HIV/AIDS
and Hepatitis:

Everything You Need to Know to
Protect Yourself and Others

HIV/AIDS and Hepatitis:

Everything You Need to Know to Protect Yourself and Others

Douglas D. Schoon

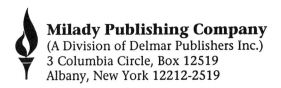

Milady Publishing Company
(A Division of Delmar Publishers Inc.)
3 Columbia Circle, Box 12519
Albany, New York 12212-2519

NOTICE TO THE READER

Credits:
Publisher: Catherine Frangie
Developmental Editor: Laura V. Miller
Art/Design Supervisor: Susan C. Mathews
Production Manager: John Mickelbank

Freelance Project Editor: Gail Hamrick

Copyright © 1994
Milady Publishing Company
(A Division of Delmar Publishers Inc.)

For information address:
Milady Publishing Company
(A Division of Delmar Publishers Inc.)
3 Columbia Circle, Box 12519
Albany, NY 12212-2519

Printed in the United States of America
Published simultaneously in Canada
by Nelson Canada
a Division of The Thomson Corporation

2 3 4 5 6 7 8 9 10 XXX 00 99 98 97 96 95

Library of Congress Cataloging-in-Publication Data

Schoon, Douglas D.
    HIV/AIDS and hepatitis : everything you need to know to protect
yourself and others / Douglas D. Schoon
        p.   cm.
    Includes bibliographical references and index.
    ISBN 1-56253-175-1
    1. AIDS (Disease)—Popular works. 2. Hepatitis—Popular works.
I. Title.
RC607.A26S3736   1994   93-27797
616.97'92—dc20   CIP

Dedication

to all the animals

On the day disease is conquered
the last virus controlled
We'll look to our past
the truth will unfold
In those first few moments
I hope we will see
It wasn't just you
It wasn't just me
...we have the animals to thank!

D. Schoon

CHAPTER SIX

CHAPTER SEVEN

APPENDIX A

APPENDIX B
Answers to
Test-Your-Knowledge

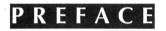

PREFACE

In the past 40 years, medical researchers have learned astounding things about the human body and its function. Over 95% of all medical and biological knowledge has been discovered since 1950! We are fortunate to be living in the golden age of biology, but rapid progress has its drawbacks as well.

Most people feel out of touch with science and medicine. Even scientists have trouble keeping up with the information explosion. Still, it is very important to learn as much as possible about new developments. Being informed is the best way to protect yourself and your loved ones. In this age of information, knowledge is the key to survival.

As a beauty industry professional, it is your duty to keep abreast of the latest information on infectious diseases. Your clients expect nothing less. Sanitation and disinfection controls are now more important than ever.

Why Read This Book?

The purpose of this book is twofold:

1. To explain, in simple terms, how to control infectious diseases.

2. To dispel the myths and eliminate the irrational fears caused by misinformation.

Although controlling all infectious diseases is the main theme, the focus of this book is on HIV/AIDS and hepatitis. You will learn what causes these diseases; how they are spread; and how to prevent infecting yourself, clients, friends, and family. You will also learn the truth, without hype or scare tactics. Unfortunately, much of what people think they know about AIDS (things they read in a magazine or saw on television) are actually overdramatized, sensationalized, distortions of the facts.

To begin with, try taking this self-test to see how informed you are about AIDS.

1. Do you think AIDS is growing among homosexuals?

2. Do you believe that the average high school student runs a great risk of getting AIDS if sexually active?

3. If dentists or doctors have AIDS, do you think they are likely to infect patients?

4. Does the average heterosexual in America have a good chance of getting AIDS?

5. Is there currently a great risk of getting AIDS from blood transfusions?

6. Do you believe everyone who has unprotected sex with someone with AIDS will eventually become infected?

7. If you touch the blood of a person with AIDS will you become infected?

8. Do you think the risk of getting AIDS is greater than the risk of getting hepatitis?

9. Do you believe that while performing your normal services there is a good chance of getting AIDS from an infected client?

10. Do you think that AIDS strikes randomly or that everyone has the same HIV infection risk?

11. Do most babies born to mothers infected with HIV (AIDS virus) become infected?

12. Should most mothers worry that their baby may get AIDS?

13. Is HIV the deadliest virus of this century?

14. From 1981 to 1993 were more than 0.1% (one tenth of a percent) of the American public diagnosed with AIDS?

If you answered yes to any one of these questions you may be suffering from ARH—AIDS-Related Hysteria. Each of these are misconceptions spread by irresponsible media reporting.

This book will answer your questions with the unbiased truth, based on the latest scientific information. You will find that many fears about HIV/AIDS are actually distortions and exaggerations intended to alarm the public.

AIDS is a widespread, terrible disease, but the risks and dangers are not as great as most Americans believe. With education, proper understanding, and valid information, each of us can do our part to stop the spread of this virus. People with AIDS need our help and sympathy, not our fear!

Some believe that only fear can motivate change. Sadly, past experience has often proven this theory to be correct. But fear is not the only way, nor is it the best way. Banishing the AIDS myths eliminates fear. Once the fear is gone from our minds, we can begin to think clearly, rationally, and intelligently. From these seeds, positive change will sprout and flourish.

Helpful Hints to Students

Learning any subject can be made easier. In many ways, going to school is like a job. The job of learning is up to each student, but there are ways to make the job easier and more enjoyable. The following advice will help you get the most from reading this book.

Although this book is designed to make it easier to learn, textbooks are not novels. You cannot expect to quickly read or skim each chapter and know everything. You must do some studying. These tips will help you learn.

1. Look for the words in *italics.*

While reading the chapters you will notice that some words are unfamiliar. Usually, these words will be highlighted in *italics*. Pay special attention to any word in *italics and make sure you understand its meaning.*

2. Use the chapter summaries as a guide.

At the end of each chapter you will find a Fast Track, or chapter summary. These summaries review the most important ideas from the chapter. Be sure to read the summaries several times. If you don't understand a topic, go back and reread that part of the chapter.

3. Teach your friends and family.

Research has shown the best way to learn a subject is to teach it to another person. Most people are concerned about HIV/AIDS and other diseases. You will find plenty of people willing to hear what you have learned. **Remember, by teaching others, you teach yourself.**

4. Don't just skip over what you don't understand.

There is no shame in asking your teacher to explain something you find difficult to understand. That's a teacher's job. Most teachers will be thrilled and impressed if you show a real interest in learning. Your future employers will see this desire to learn, as well. Nobody wants to hire people who think they know it all or have closed minds. Learn for the rest of your life! What you know can shape your future, even save your life.

❏ **Note**

This text contains footnotes and end-of-chapter reference notes. Footnotes are referenced with **letters** and appear at the foot of the page. End-of-chapter notes are referenced with **numbers** and appear at the end of each chapter.

ABOUT THE AUTHOR

Douglas Schoon obtained his master's degree in chemistry from the University of California—Irvine. He has more than 20 years of experience as a chemical researcher, lecturer, and educator. He is the president and founder of the Chemical Awareness Training Service, based in Newport Beach, California. Mr. Schoon has authored dozens of articles and lectured nationwide on the important topic of salon chemical safety.

As a research consultant for leading manufacturers, Mr. Schoon has developed many successful professional products for the beauty industry. He also serves as an expert witness in legal cases helping attorneys, judges, and juries to understand the chemical complexities of professional and retail beauty industry products.

Mr. Schoon is a member of the Nail Manufacturer's Council's Safety and Standards Committee (a division of the American Beauty Association), which is concerned with disinfection and sanitation safety and methods, as well as chemical safety.

ACKNOWLEDGMENTS

I would like to express my deepest gratitude to Corrine Dillard and Judy Landis-Storm. This book benefited greatly from their keen insights and valuable suggestions.

I would also like to thank the following people for their assistance and expertise in preparing and reviewing the final manuscript.

Patrick J. Furlong, M.S., Ph.D.
Oxnard, California

Victoria Peters
Nails Magazine
Torrance, California

Robert Reed
Hikari Products, Inc.
Gardena, California

Gerri Cevetillo
Ultronics, Inc.
New York, New York

Jack Wagner
Micro-Aseptic Products, Inc.
Palatine, Illinois

Jan Daughenbaugh
Fullerton College
Fullerton, California

Stacy Sloan
Creative Nail Design, Inc.
Carlsbad, California

Sidney Bane
Creative Nail Design, Inc.
Carlsbad, California

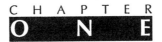
The Origins of HIV and AIDS

In May 1981, Sandra Ford, a technician at the Center for Disease Control (CDC) in Atlanta, Georgia, noticed something very peculiar. Ms. Ford's job was to keep track of orders for drugs used to treat rare diseases. One day she noticed there had been five requests for a special medicine in less than eight months. This special medicine was used to treat an extremely rare type of pneumonia and was so rarely used it had been needed only twice before in the last 12 years. She thought it strange there were five requests in only eight months, so Ms. Ford brought the matter to the attention of her supervisor. On that spring morning Ms. Ford became the first person to discover clues of the AIDS epidemic.

Following up on Ms. Ford's discovery, a group of medical specialists learned that all five requests for this drug were from Los Angeles. Also, in every case the patient was a young, male homosexual. Further investigations uncovered other interesting facts. Over a 30-month period there had been 26 cases of **Kaposi's sarcoma** (ka-**PO**-seez sar-**KO**-mah), an extremely rare form of cancer. Again, homosexual men in California, as well as New York, were the victims.

After an intense scientific study it was determined that a new disease had appeared. The disease seemed to break down the body's natural defenses, allowing other infections and cancers to spread unchecked. The disease was called ***AIDS—acquired immune deficiency syndrome*** (also ***acquired immunodeficiency syndrome***).

What is AIDS?

AIDS is actually a syndrome, not a disease. A ***syndrome*** is a collection of signs and symptoms that warn of a disease. For example, sore throat, fever, and aching joints are a collection of symptoms that warn that you may be coming down with the flu.

Each of us is born with an incredible, built-in defense system that protects our health around the clock. It is called the ***immune system***. More will be said about the immune system and how it protects us in chapter 3. For now, it is important to understand that this is how we stay healthy.

When something goes wrong with the immune system, the body loses its natural ability to fight infection and disease. If this were to happen to a previously healthy person, he or she would have acquired an ***immune deficiency*** (lack of a properly functioning immune system). The collection of signs and symptoms that occur in such a case is called acquired immune deficiency syndrome or AIDS. Usually you will see the second and third word placed together to make immunodeficiency. Either way, the meaning is the same.

Now you can see that AIDS is not a disease. It is a collection of symptoms that show that the body is no longer capable of protecting itself from infection or disease. You can't catch a syndrome; therefore you can't "catch" AIDS.

HIV—The Cause of AIDS

What causes a person to acquire an immune deficiency like AIDS? It is caused by a tiny, invisible virus called ***HIV—human immunodeficiency virus*** (Figure 1-1). A ***virus*** is different from a bacteria. Viruses are much smaller and simpler. Viruses are so simple they cannot live or reproduce on their own. To live, a virus must *infect* a bacteria or tissue cell. More will be said about viruses in the next chapter.

FIGURE 1–1
HIV (AIDS-causing virus) as seen under a powerful electron microscope. *(From: VIRUSES by A.J. Levine. Copyright © 1991 by W.H. Freeman and Company. Reprinted by permission.)*

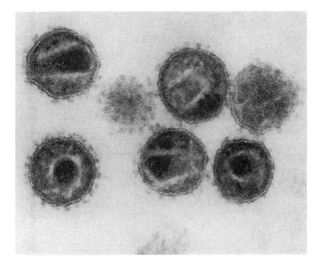

Where Did HIV Come From?

There have been many theories about HIV and where it came from. Africans see the disease as a product of Western lifestyles. A popular myth in the country Zaire is that the virus arrived from the United States in a shipment of army surplus clothing. More paranoid theories from other parts of the world claim that the virus was created in secret military laboratories.

The last idea is probably the most foolish of all. For over 11 years, thousands of the world's best scientists have been feverishly working to unravel the secrets of HIV. Only now are they beginning to fully understand how HIV spreads and reproduces. For HIV to have been created, a scientist would have had to know more about viruses in the fifties than all of the scientists' combined knowledge of the nineties. The idea is utterly ridiculous.

One reason for so many silly notions about the beginnings of AIDS is that discovering the original source of HIV was not an easy task for scientists. For many years, the issue was widely disputed, but in 1990 Beatrice Hahn and George Shaw, two scientists at the University of Alabama, made an important discovery. They learned that one type of HIV is almost identical to a virus found in the African green monkey. After this important finding was reported, special studies on how HIV has evolved (changed over time) indicated that HIV has existed for at least 40 years.

Further evidence has also been uncovered to support this idea. Stored, frozen blood samples taken from people in Africa in 1959 contained the AIDS-causing virus, HIV.

Why Did the AIDS Epidemic Happen?

Many lessons can be learned from history. Great epidemics have often occurred because of sudden social, political, or economic changes. The smallpox virus was brought to the New World by a small band of Spanish explorers in 1520. Yellow fever virus (also found in wild animals) escaped from Africa on slave trading ships in the seventeenth century. The syphilis virus was also spread around the world by early seafaring travelers.

Researchers now believe that the AIDS virus may have existed in Africa for many years. Monkeys are used for food in rural parts of Africa. Hunters were probably infected through small cuts on their hands while cleaning infected meat or scraping hides for clothing. The disease may have reoccurred and died out many times in these small villages, never going any further.

But in the late fifties, Africa began to grow quickly. Large cities and urban centers literally sprang from the jungle. This caused a drastic change in the traditional way of life for Africans. The sudden appearance of highly populated areas started the spread of HIV.

This would explain why Africa has been hardest hit by the AIDS epidemic. The World Health Organization (WHO) estimates that in the nineties over 80% of all AIDS cases in the world will occur in central Africa.[1] The virus has probably been slowly spreading there undetected for many decades, possibly centuries.

What Are the Real Risks?

High risks, low risks, great risks, no risks—what does it all mean? The media is constantly bombarding us with stories about the risks of being infected with the AIDS virus, but they rarely seem to give any solid facts. Scientific estimates about the risks are usually misunderstood by both the media and the general public. The result has been chaos and confusion. Statistics are often used to mislead and frighten people, and AIDS statistics and information have been no exception.

Before we can begin to understand the risks, we must first define the word. Scientists define **risk** as the possibility of injury or death. When scientists make an estimate or calculation of the risks, it is called **risk assessment**.

Risk Assessment

Imagine the following situation. What would you do if you were told that behind Door #1 there was one million dollars in cash? All you had to do was open the door and it would be yours, tax free! Of course, anyone would open the door.

Now suppose you were told that there was a one in three chance you would be struck by lightning and killed instantly when you opened the door. Only the very daring or desperate would open that door.

But what if the risk of being struck by lightning was only 1 in 50? Of course, more people would take the chance.

How about if the risks were changed to 1 in 1,000? Probably a lot of people would think these were good odds and open the door. What about 1 in 200,000? Very few people would pass up this opportunity. Still, a few people might say no until the amount was raised to ten million dollars.

This exercise was more than just a simple game of fantasy. You have been making a risk assessment—examining the likelihood of being injured or killed, then deciding if it is worth the risk. You do this every day without realizing it. If you walk, drive, ride the train, or take the bus to work each day you are taking a risk. If you drive, you have decided the risk of being injured or killed in a car is small compared to the benefits of driving.

It would be impossible to live without taking any chances. When a mother lets her child receive a shot of penicillin for a bad throat infection, she is accepting the 1 in 100,000 chance that the child may go into shock and possibly die. Sure it's possible, but she realizes that the benefit far exceeds the risk.

Slightly more than half of all high school and college football players are injured each year.[2] Some of these injuries result in serious or permanent disabilities. Should we ban the sport from schools? Most would say no. However, if half the players were killed each year the game would certainly be prohibited as the risks would outweigh the benefits.

Life is a gamble. If you're not prepared to take certain risks, you're not prepared for life. Table 1–1 shows some commonly accepted risks Americans are willing to take each day.

Table 1–1: Worth the Risks?

Odds of being killed by a dog	1 in 700,000
Odds of being killed in a car accident	1 in 125
Odds of being killed in a bicycle accident	1 in 200,000
Odds of being killed in a plane accident	1 in 4,600,000
Odds of being injured on the job	1 in 61
Odds of being attacked by a shark	1 in 2,000,000
Odds of being injured by lightning	1 in 9,100
Odds of getting skin cancer	1 in 460
Odds of getting cancer from side stream smoke	1 in 40,000
Odds that you will regain all weight loss after a diet	9 in 10

(*Source:* What the Odds Are, *Les Krantz, Harper-Perennial, 1992*)

Sure there is a chance that the airplane you are flying in will crash. Wouldn't it be silly to avoid flying at all simply because there was a 1 in 4,600,000 chance? You're safer flying than driving a car. You are 36,800 times more likely to be killed in a car accident. Flying is even safer than riding a bike!

Taking Risks

Air transportation is a marvelous, modern-day convenience. Still, many people needlessly avoid flying and travel by the more dangerous routes. Why? They misunderstand the true risks.

It is important to understand the true meaning of the word *risk*. Just because there is a risk or a chance of something happening does not mean it will happen. For example, there is a chance that a huge asteroid will crash into the Earth next month. So should we all quit working, take an around-the-world vacation, and run up our credit cards?

Common sense says you should control and lower risks, not live in fear! With knowledge you can control risks. The more you know, the easier it is to protect yourself. Not being properly informed can cause you to do the wrong thing and increase your risks, instead of lowering them. Driving to New York from California is far riskier than flying, not safer.

HIV/AIDS Risks in America

You don't have to look far to find a story about HIV or AIDS. Both are popular topics with newspapers, magazines, radio, and television. Next time you run across a story pay close attention. Do they ever give any real information about HIV infection risks?

Typically you'll read or hear statements like, "AIDS cases increased by 10% over last year" or "the number of cases is growing at epidemic proportion." What do these two statements have in common? Neither tells us anything at all. They are intended to shock or frighten, not provide useful information.

The Media Strikes Out

The American media is easily the most irresponsible news organization in the world.[a] The media pretends to

---

a. In the opinion of the author.

"educate" Americans about AIDS, but they have failed us miserably.

In recent years, the media has become big business. Increased ratings are now all that is important. Media executives know they can increase their ratings with stories about violent crimes, riots, wars, disease, catastrophes, and disasters. People are more likely to pay attention to these types of stories, and increased ratings means more money.

So, as the networks battle for your attention, you are constantly bombarded with more and more shocking stories. Ratings increase even higher when these stories are exaggerated or dramatized. HIV- and AIDS-related stories are certainly no exception. Usually, AIDS "stories" are based on inaccurate estimates, which are then presented completely out of perspective. Why? To frighten the public and increase profits.

Scientific Estimates

Scientists make estimations about the spread of HIV to help the government and health care organizations plan for the future. The media sensationalizes their reports and pretends that these scientific "guesses" are scientific facts that are bound to occur.

Oftentimes, reporters aren't really "reporting" but are giving their uninformed opinions. The majority are trained in journalism, not science. Reporters automatically interpret AIDS stories with negative attitudes. They then represent their own interpretations as if they were facts.

Unfortunately, many people have been misled! Many believe things are probably even worse than what scientists and the government are telling us. Actually, the opposite is true. The government and scientists have consistently **overestimated** the severity of the AIDS epidemic in the United States.

Scientific and Government AIDS Predictions

The first government prediction concerning the spread of AIDS in America was made in 1986. The Public Health Service predicted that by the end of 1991 the total number of reported AIDS cases would be 270,000. They were wrong! This prediction was much too high. The actual count turned out to be 34% lower (179,136 reported cases instead of 270,000).

In 1988, this same government agency raised the predictions to 365,000 total reported AIDS cases by the end of 1992. Again, these predictions were too high. The actual figure was 253,448, or 30% lower than predicted.

In 1989, a group of top government AIDS experts and other scientists predicted that in 1990 there would be between 52,000 and 57,000 new cases reported.[3] The actual number turned out to be about 20% lower than even their most conservative estimate.

Government predictions are only estimates. They are never accurate. Usually the number of reported AIDS cases is far less than the prediction. Still, the media never fails to suggest that the real number of cases is even higher than predicted. These rough estimates spawned dozens of reports and articles during the eighties with titles like "AIDS: At the Dawn of Fear" (I think you can see where they're headed with this title). If you read these articles today, they seem almost comical. They are filled with dire warnings of a gloomy future without much hope. Very few of these fearful exaggerations have actually come true.

What Is the Truth?

The real facts about HIV and AIDS are not rosy. Many innocent people have died and many more will follow. But the situation is not nearly as bad as most believe. AIDS is not everywhere. The media has been telling us only half the truth, the bad half. If America is truly on "The Dawn of Fear," it isn't because of AIDS. We can blame the American mass media and their greed.

There is a lot of good news about HIV and AIDS. The future is not as bleak as you may have heard.

AIDS in Perspective

Looking at the facts in *perspective* means to see the whole picture or how the facts compare with other similar ideas. It is easy to be fooled by figures if you don't look at them properly. We must always view statistics and facts in perspective, so that we can see their real importance. For example, imagine what you would think if you heard the following special report on television:

> Today, scientists reported that by using a newly developed technique they can measure chemical contamination in food much more accurately than ever before. In the same report these scientists claim to have used this technique to test every type of baby food on the market.

> They discovered that each baby food tested contained detectable amounts of lead, a chemical known to be extremely toxic and capable of causing cancer. A government spokesperson reluctantly admitted that the report was accurate, but defended the lack of action by saying, "...we're not surprised at the findings. A special panel was appointed to look into the matter and saw no need for concern."

Obviously, a report such as this would cause widespread panic. People would be not only shocked that baby food was contaminated, but angry that the government wasn't doing something about the problem. However, the facts have not been presented "in perspective" (a common news media tactic). This same story, presented in perspective, would not be frightening at all.

Scientists use highly sophisticated instruments capable of measuring extremely small amounts of chemicals. Present technology allows measurements of one part per billion (1ppb), i.e. one molecule of salt diluted in one billion molecules of water. Lead is a substance found in nature. Lead can probably be found everywhere. Lead is potentially dangerous at high concentrations, but is harmless in extremely small amounts—even in baby food. The reporter didn't mention that it would probably be impossible to find any food that had absolutely zero lead. This story shows that you can make anything sound bad—if you leave out the right information.

By not telling the viewer that very small amounts of lead are safe, the reporter presented the facts out of perspective. Now you can see why it is so important to always look at things in perspective. Usually, the facts are much less frightening when they are properly presented.

If HIV/AIDS statistics are examined in their proper perspective, without the media hype and scare tactics, you can see that AIDS is an easily avoided disease. We'll look at all the facts and then examine the risks.

HIV/AIDS Statistics

You have probably never seen a map like the one shown in Figure 1-2. This map shows the total number of AIDS cases reported between 1981 and 1992. (Federal law requires that all cases of AIDS be reported.) It is probably not surprising to find that reported AIDS cases seem to be concentrated on the East and West coasts. States like Montana, Nebraska, North and South Dakota, Idaho, and Wyoming have reported relatively few cases.

Even though this map is correct, it too can be deceiving. The highest numbers of reported cases seem to be in New York, California, Florida, Texas, and New Jersey. But, it is

FIGURE 1–2
Total number of AIDS cases reported to the Center for Disease Control (CDC) by January 1, 1993. *(Source: CDC Wonder Database, April 1993)*

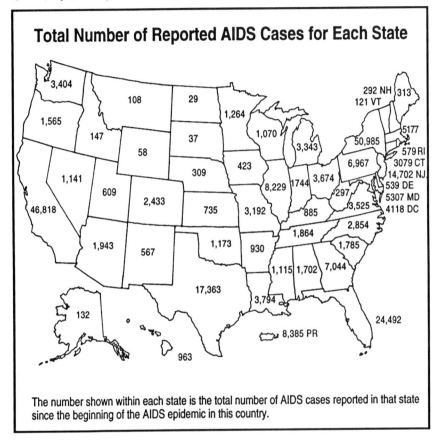

Total Number of Reported AIDS Cases for Each State

The number shown within each state is the total number of AIDS cases reported in that state since the beginning of the AIDS epidemic in this country.

important to account for the population of each state as the next map shows.

Figure 1-3 on page 14 shows the same map, but the number of reported AIDS cases has been adjusted by state population. These numbers show how many reported cases of AIDS there are for every 100,000 people, and they tell quite a different story.

When the population is considered, the picture changes. Washington, D.C. has the highest rate of reported AIDS

FIGURE 1–3

Number of AIDS cases per 100,000 inhabitants reported to the Center for
Disease Control (CDC) by January 1, 1993. *(Source: CDC Wonder
Database, April 1993)*

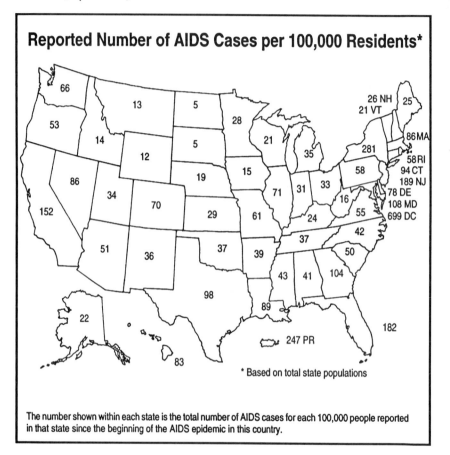

Reported Number of AIDS Cases per 100,000 Residents*

* Based on total state populations

The number shown within each state is the total number of AIDS cases for each 100,000 people reported
in that state since the beginning of the AIDS epidemic in this country.

cases per 100,000 residents followed by New York, New Jersey, Puerto Rico, and Florida. California and Texas are no
longer in the top five. Note that Figure 1-2 incorrectly sug-
gests that Washington, D.C. has a lower disease rate than
neighboring Maryland when it is actually six and one-half
times higher than Maryland.

These maps not only show the importance of looking at statistics in perspective, they also provide information about

risks of exposure. Clearly, people living in North Dakota have a far lower risk than those living in Washington, D.C. or New York City. Where you live can help determine your risk of being infected with HIV.

Children with AIDS—Should Mothers Be Afraid?

Another way the media has manipulated the public is by suggesting there is a terrible AIDS threat to children and teens. If this is true, there must certainly be cause for alarm. Once again, let's examine the truth—in perspective.

Figure 1-4 shows that AIDS cases among children were only 1.7% of all reported AIDS cases between 1981 and 1992.

FIGURE 1–4
The total number and percent of children diagnosed with AIDS from 1981 to 1992. The majority of these children (3,665 or 86%) were originally infected by HIV-positive mothers. *(Source: CDC cumulative statistics up to December 1992)*

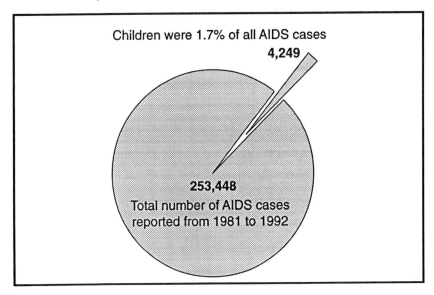

Children were 1.7% of all AIDS cases
4,249

253,448
Total number of AIDS cases
reported from 1981 to 1992

Sadly, 86% (3,665) of these children with AIDS were infected by HIV-positive mothers. The overwhelming majority of these mothers injected illegal drugs or had partners who were infected by sharing HIV-contaminated needles. About 12% were infected by blood transfusions during the early days of the epidemic. Infections are rarely caused by blood transfusions now as blood banks and hospitals carefully test all blood for HIV before it is used.

Of course, even one child with AIDS is a terrible thing. At first glance, 4,249 children with AIDS may seem like a frighteningly large number. But look again, to be sure you are understanding the truth of the situation.

These statistics show that the number of children who have AIDS is actually very small. About 4 million babies are born in the United States each year; therefore, approximately 44 million babies were born between 1981 and 1992. This means that only about 50 in every 1 million babies have gotten AIDS since 1981.

This doesn't mean that 50 babies in a million is acceptable. It does mean that a baby is highly unlikely to get AIDS (1 in 20,000). The truth is, mothers who do not inject drugs have a nearly zero chance that their baby will be infected with HIV. Even in mothers who are HIV positive, only one in three babies becomes infected.

It is sad that any young child should have to suffer with AIDS. But Americans are quite lucky. In Asia, Latin America, and Africa 4.6 million children under the age of five die each year from ***viral gastroenteritis*** (gas-tro-en-ta-**RYE**-tis), a fatal type of diarrhea. More children die each year in these countries from diarrhea than are born in the United States.

Teen AIDS—Is Our Youth in Danger?

There has been a great deal of debate on the subject of educating teens about AIDS. Should the schools or family be responsible? What should the government be doing?

These debates are likely to continue for some time with no clear answers.

Education is the key to stopping the spread of HIV. The gay community proved this by drastically reducing the rate of HIV infection and AIDS among homosexuals. This was done primarily through intensive and positive education.

Unfortunately, much of the education aimed at teens is designed to frighten them out of having sex, rather than educate them about avoiding AIDS. Many groups have seized the opportunity created by the AIDS epidemic to preach their views of morality, instead of teaching the facts. Let's look at the facts once again. Do America's teens have a high risk of being infected with HIV?

Figure 1–5 shows the total number of reported teen AIDS cases in the United States. There are an estimated 14

FIGURE 1–5

Total number of AIDS cases reported among teenagers between 1981 and 1992. *(CDC Statistics)*

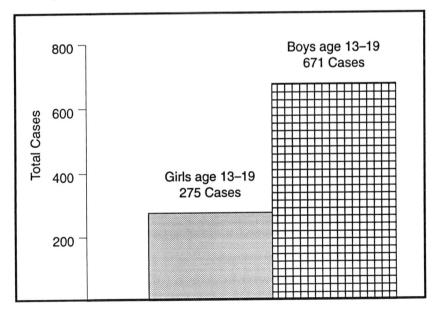

million high school students (grades 9–12) in the United States. According to the Center for Disease Control (CDC), between 1981 and 1993, 275 teenage girls and 671 teenage boys were diagnosed with AIDS. Surprisingly, only 136 teenagers (12 males and 124 females) have developed AIDS through heterosexual (male/female) sex. Of the remaining 810 cases reported to the CDC, 122 were caused by injecting drugs and sharing needles, 265 were in homosexual and bisexual males,[b] 339 were related to blood products or transfusions, and 14 were in teens born in other countries. The remaining 70 cases had undetermined causes. Figure 1–6 illustrates this breakdown of causes for the reported cases of AIDS in teens.

In 1988, over 7,200 teenagers died in automobile accidents. A survey made in 1991 found that the suicide rate among 15–19 year olds quadrupled between 1950 and 1988.[4] In 1989, 276,000 high school students in the United States made at least one suicide attempt that required medical attention. One in every 12 American children will run away from home before turning 18. According to the Surgeon General's Survey on Alcoholism, two in five teens drink weekly and one in four of these are classified as alcoholics.

AIDS is a problem that must be dealt with in the schools, but it is not the only problem, nor is it the biggest or most serious problem facing America's youth. Educating teens about AIDS will obviously have great long-term benefits, helping them cope with drugs, alcohol, and depression will have even greater benefits.

Clearly, young people have many other important problems that must not be forgotten or pushed aside. We cannot win the war against AIDS by fearing it.

---

b. According to the CDC, no known cases of AIDS have ever occurred between gay females (lesbians).

FIGURE 1–6
Most common reported cause of AIDS in American teenagers between
1981 and 1992. *(CDC Statistics)*

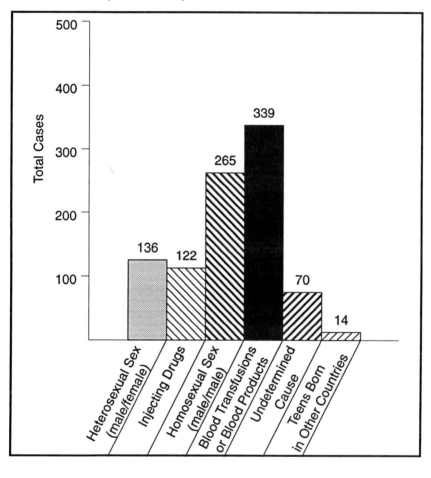

Irrational Fear

In 1987 the American Medical Association (AMA) con-
ducted a survey that found that 50% of Americans believed that AIDS was very likely to kill a large share of the
population.[5] There is absolutely no scientific evidence to
support this belief. The AMA said in October of the following year, "...AIDS is not 'exploding' into the heterosexual

population relative to other risk groups."[6] Then why is the public so afraid?

After 11 years of the epidemic, 0.1% (one-tenth of a percent) of the United States population have been diagnosed with AIDS. After 11 years, only 1–2% of the homosexuals in the United States have AIDS, and they are in one of the highest risk categories. The truth is, many experts believe that the AIDS rate is slowing in many high-risk categories in the United States. Clearly, the media could do more to calm these irrational fears.

The world is not a perfect place to live. Everyone knows that! Despite all our knowledge, people get sick. Humans are fragile beings. Ten million people a year die from pneumonia. Eight thousand people die each week from heart disease in the United States alone. During the first 11 years of the AIDS epidemic 172,000 people have died from AIDS. But consider this; in that same period **almost three times as many women have died from breast cancer.**

In 1900, infectious diseases were the leading cause of death in the United States, causing nearly 37% of all deaths. In 1989, only 2.8% of all deaths were caused by infectious diseases.

Without question, AIDS is a terrible disease. But remember that there are many far worse risks in the world. How is it that we have learned to accept these other far greater risks? By seeing them in their proper perspective.

What You Will Learn

In the following chapters, you will learn that AIDS is not a fearful monster that randomly infects the unsuspecting. HIV is not running wild through our schools. Most people in America have little risk of being infected with HIV. In fact, you'll discover it's quite easy to lower your risk of infection to nearly zero.

You will also discover that there are still many other infectious diseases in the world. The media focuses on HIV/AIDS, but other diseases are far more likely to visit your salon. But never fear, just as with HIV, it is easy to protect yourself and prevent the spread of disease. That is one of the basic responsibilities of your profession.

❑ FAST TRACK

1. The first clues of AIDS were discovered in May 1981 by Sandra Ford, a technician at the Center for Disease Control (CDC) in Atlanta, Georgia.

2. Homosexuals in New York and California were becoming ill with an extremely rare type of pneumonia and Kaposi's sarcoma, an extremely rare form of cancer.

3. AIDS stands for "acquired immunodeficiency syndrome."

4. AIDS is a syndrome, not a disease.

5. A syndrome is a collection of signs and symptoms that warn of a disease.

6. When something goes wrong with the immune system, the body loses its natural ability to fight infection and disease.

7. You can't catch a syndrome; therefore you can't "catch" AIDS.

8. AIDS is caused by a tiny, invisible virus called HIV (human immunodeficiency virus).

9. Viruses are so simple they cannot live or reproduce on their own; they must infect a bacteria or tissue cell.

10. Scientists now believe that HIV originated in Africa more than 40 years ago.

11. Great epidemics often occurred because of sudden social, political, or economic changes.

12. Smallpox, yellow fever, and syphilis are examples of viruses spread by sea travelers.

13. In the late fifties, large cities grew in Africa, starting the spread of HIV.

14. The World Health Organization (WHO) estimates that in the nineties over 80% of all AIDS cases in the world will occur in central Africa.

15. Scientists define *risk* as the possibility of injury or death.

16. Scientific estimates or calculation of the risks is called risk assessment.

17. It would be impossible to live without taking any risks or chances. Life is a gamble.

18. Common sense says we should control and lower risks, not live in fear!

19. The mass media presents distorted views about AIDS in the United States and the world.

20. The government and scientists have consistently over-estimated the severity of the AIDS epidemic.

21. It is important to view facts in perspective—to see the whole picture or how the facts compare with other similar ideas.

22. During the first 11 years of the epidemic (1981–1992) children accounted for only 1.7% of all reported AIDS cases. The majority (86%) of these children with AIDS were infected by HIV-positive mothers and fathers who became infected by sharing HIV-contaminated needles.

23. Infections are now rarely caused by blood transfusions.

24. In Asia, Latin America, and Africa, 4.6 million children under the age of five die each year from viral gastroenteritis, a fatal type of diarrhea.

25. During the first 11 years of the epidemic (1981–1992), 275 teenage girls and 671 teenage boys were reported to have AIDS. Of these, only 136 teenagers (out of approximately 14 million total high school students) developed AIDS through heterosexual (male/female) sex.

26. After 11 years of the epidemic, 0.1% (one-tenth of a percent) of the United States population has been reported to have developed AIDS.

27. After 11 years of the epidemic only 1–2% of the homo-sexuals in the United States have been diagnosed with AIDS, and they are in one of the highest risk categories.

28. Many experts believe that the AIDS rate is slowing in many high-risk categories in the United States.

29. There are many other infectious diseases far more likely to visit your salon than HIV/AIDS.

30. It is easy to protect yourself and prevent the spread of disease.

❏ TEST YOUR KNOWLEDGE

Answers are in Appendix B.

1. In what year were the first clues of the AIDS epidemic discovered?

2. AIDS stands for _____   _____
   _____   _____.

3. What is the name of the virus that causes AIDS?

4. Where does the World Health Organization predict that over 80% of all AIDS cases in the nineties will occur?

5. Looking at the whole picture or how the facts compare with other similar ideas is called using proper
   _____.

6. What percentage to the United States population has been diagnosed with AIDS in the first 11 years of the epidemic?

7. Children make up about ___% of all AIDS cases.

8. True or False
   According to the statistics presented in this chapter, HIV is not likely to infect a large portion of Americans.

❏ REFERENCE NOTES

1. *UN Chronicle, 27* (4), (1990, December), p. 66.

2. Vinger, P. F., & Hoerner, E. F. (1982). *Sports Injuries: The Unthwarted Epidemic.*

3. *Journal of the American Medical Association (JAMA), 262* (11), (1990, March 16), p. 1477.

4. *JAMA, 266* (14), (1991, October 9), p. 1911.

5. Doctor, R. M. & Kahn, A. P. *The Encyclopedia of Phobias, Fears and Anxieties* (p. 2). Facts on File, New York: Oxford.

6. *AIDS Reference Guide (113),* (1988, November), Atlantic Information Services, Inc.

T W O

Transmitting the AIDS Virus

Our bodies are made up of many different organs. The organs are arranged into systems that work for the benefit of the whole being. Without mutual cooperation and organization, higher forms of life could not exist.

For example, the ***respiratory system*** is made up of the mouth, throat, windpipe, and lungs. This system carries oxygen from the outside environment to the blood and removes carbon dioxide.

Another example is the ***circulatory system***, consisting of the heart, arteries, veins, and capillaries. This system pumps blood to the other organs of the body. Many such systems work together to maintain a healthy body.

Each individual organ is also a group or system of many smaller ***cells***. The kidney is made of millions of kidney cells; the heart is made up of many heart cells. Plants are also made of cells. Plant cells are similar in many ways to those found in the human body.

In general, biologists define a cell as the smallest and simplest unit capable of being alive. In this respect, human liver or kidney cells are remarkably similar to amoebas (microscopic, one-celled creatures found in rivers or pond water) or bacteria. All cells bring in food and use it to make substances necessary for life and reproduction.

The Microscopic World

Plant cells are the largest type of cell, but even they must be magnified to be clearly visible. Plant cells are about four ten-thousandths of an inch in diameter. Animal cells are 10 times smaller. Bacteria are 100 times smaller (see Table 2–1). Because of their extremely small size, bacteria are called microorganisms (micro meaning small, and organism meaning living creature).

Bacteria are the smallest microorganisms capable of making their own energy and reproducing. They are like tiny factories. The human body and bacteria have much in common. Both contain many internal organs. Of course, bacteria don't have stomachs, livers, and hearts, but they have other organs that do similar jobs, such as transporting food and sorting and removing waste products. They also build proteins and other useful substances the bacteria needs to grow and reproduce.

Reproduction is another important way bacteria resemble humans. Bacteria reproduce or make copies of themselves. They do this in the same way humans do. No, bacteria don't turn down the lights, put on quiet music, and sip

TABLE 2–1:   Sizes of Microscopic Cells and Particles Compared to the Diameter of Hair

Cell or Particle	Size (inches)	Compared to Hair
Human Hair	0.004	
Plant Cells	0.002 5	1.6 times smaller
Animal Cells	0.000 4	10 times smaller
Bacteria	0.000 04	100 times smaller
Viruses	0.000 000 8	5,000 times smaller
Proteins	0.000 000 2	20,000 times smaller
Amino Acids	0.000 000 03	133,000 times smaller
Atoms	0.000 000 001	4,000,000 times smaller

champagne, but they do use another of our secrets of reproduction—DNA.

The Source of Life

If we didn't have a way of making nearly exact copies of ourselves, the human race would die out quickly. Fortunately, all living things, from humans to bacteria, carry a complete blueprint for duplicating themselves. In fact, every cell in the body carries a complete set of these blueprints, called **DNA** (stands for **deoxyribonucleic** [dee-**AHK**-see-rye-boh-new-klee-ik] **acid**).

DNA is a very special and tiny molecule that carries all of the information needed to create an exact copy of you. It is much like a computer tape, and holds billions of pieces of coded information about your eye color, and how many fingers and toes you have, as well as their exact shape, length, and location.

When DNA is observed under a very high-power microscope, it looks like two long flowing strands of ribbon, twisting around each other like spiral staircases (Figure 2–1). In humans, these strands are over six feet long. Amazingly, DNA is so tightly coiled up, it easily fits inside

FIGURE 2–1
A small section of a DNA molecule.

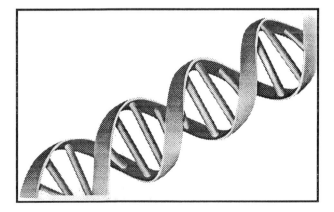

a single cell. Sticking off the ribbons are amino acids. These are the same amino acids that make up hair, skin, and nails.

Nature's Alphabet

The amino acids are arranged in a certain order on the DNA ribbons. The arrangement is like an alphabet. This alphabet is a how-to-reproduce manual for the cells. Special parts of the cell can read this "manual" and follow the instructions.

These amino acid arrangements spell out a code called the **genetic code**. The genetic code determines among other things whether you will have blue eyes or brown, long legs or short. Each one of your cells carries a full copy of your DNA code, but each cell uses only the part it needs to create a new cell. For example, your blood contains about 27.5 trillion red blood cells. The average life span for a red blood cell is 120 days. Therefore, your body must make approximately 76 billion new red blood cells each day. How can the body make so many copies of the same cell? Each duplicate cell is created from the information stored in DNA. This is similar to making many copies of the same photo from one negative.

Bacteria carry the same DNA that humans do, the only difference being that bacteria's DNA gives directions for making more bacteria. All living things—trees, insects, rodents, birds, fish, dogs—use DNA to reproduce.

Whatever your beliefs about life, it is awesome to realize that every creature, from the simplest to the most complex, uses the same DNA to carry on its existence. Certainly, DNA can be considered the source of life.

How Are Viruses Different?

At the end of the seventeenth century, a curious Dutch cloth merchant named Antony van Leeuwenhoek (Figure 2-2) got a very strange idea. Simple microscopes had recently been invented. Leeuwenhoek bought one to examine the quality

FIGURE 2–2
Antony van Leeuwenhoek (1632–1723).
(From: VIRUSES *by A.J. Levine. Copyright ©
1987 by W.H. Freeman and Company. Reprinted
by permission.)*

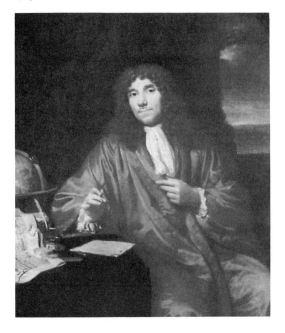

and textures of the fabrics he sold. He began to wonder
how other things would look under the microscope. Leeuwenhoek started to examine all sorts of everyday objects.
When he looked at river water he was amazed!

In a series of letters to the Royal Society of London (the
leading scientists of Europe), he described the "wee animalcules" that he saw. "...I must confess," he wrote, "that the
whole stuff seemed to me to be alive. ...the number of
these animalcules was so extraordinarily great that 'twould
take a thousand million of some of 'em to make up the bulk
of a course grain of sand."

What Leeuwenhoek saw were actually amoeba and other
types of the very largest microscopic creatures. His crude

microscope didn't have enough magnifying power to see bacteria, unlike microscopes of today (Figure 2–3).

FIGURE 2–3
This scientist uses a powerful electron microscope to see viruses. *(Photo courtesy of Carl Zeiss, Inc.)*

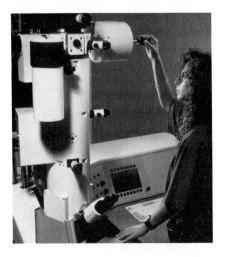

Smaller Than Bacteria

As Table 2–1 (page 26) shows, bacteria are 100 times smaller than the diameter of a human hair. Viruses, however, are 50 times smaller than bacteria. Viruses are very strange things. They are like shadows, existing between the world of the living and nonliving. They are almost alive. Viruses are too simple to make their own energy or reproduce. They need help to live.

Viruses are parasites. They can only live inside another cell called a **host cell**. Outside the host cell, viruses die quickly. Many are so delicate, they are destroyed within minutes. Studies show that 99% of HIV is destroyed after several hours on dry surfaces.[1] Though small and fragile, viruses have managed to cause humanity much grief and suffering.

History of Viruses

Even though viruses have been around as long as bacteria, scientists didn't discover them until about 100 years ago. In 1892, a young Russian scientist named Dimitrii Ivanovsky was the first to discover the existence of viruses (Figure 2–4). Eight years later, scientists learned that human diseases could be caused by viruses.

FIGURE 2–4
The first virus ever discovered was the Tobacco Mosaic Virus (as seen under an electron microscope). This virus was discovered by Russian scientist Dimitrii Ivanovsky in 1892. *(Photo courtesy of Carl Zeiss, Inc.)*

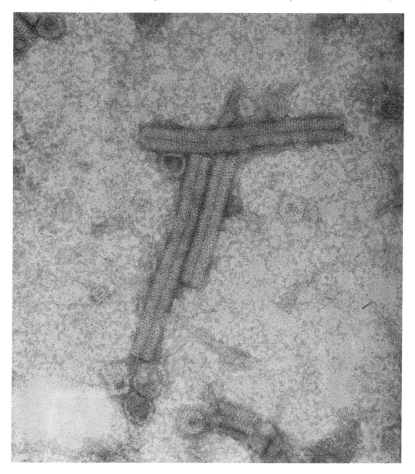

Viruses (Figure 2-5) cause many human illnesses, such as chicken pox, smallpox, influenza (flu), measles, mumps, rubella, rabies, typhoid fever, yellow fever, cold sores, herpes, AIDS, hepatitis, warts, polio, and certain kinds of cancer. At least 30 different viruses can cause the symptoms of a common cold.

How Viruses Spread

Since viruses are parasites, they must invade or infect other cells. Once the virus infects a host cell, it can grow and reproduce. Viruses are very fragile. The more delicate the virus, the more difficult it is to spread. Obviously, a virus that passes easily from one person to another is more likely to be transmitted. This is what makes a virus contagious.

Influenza (flu) viruses spread easily in tiny droplets caused by coughing or sneezing. When these droplets are inhaled or enter the mouth, the flu virus also enters and infects cells. The virus then begins to reproduce and spread. Flu viruses can also be transmitted by kissing or by touching infected surfaces. Other viruses may be spread by drinking contaminated water, for example, hepatitis A and polio.

A few viruses may be passed on by insects or animal bites. Yellow fever is transmitted by mosquito bites. Bubonic plague virus is transmitted by fleas. Contrary to popular belief, dogs rarely transmit rabies virus. Bites from bats, foxes, skunks, and cats are more likely to spread rabies.

How Viruses Grow

Once the virus enters the body it infects a tissue cell. Viruses usually prefer certain types of cells. For instance, rabies infects brain cells and chicken pox virus infects the skin. Luckily, not all types of viruses cause disease. Some infect the cells of their choice and remain in the body unnoticed, without causing sickness, disease, or damage.

Once a cell is infected by a virus many things can happen. Flu and common cold viruses reproduce rapidly. These viruses

FIGURE 2–5
Virus highly magnified under a microscope. *(Photo courtesy of Carl Zeiss, Inc.)*

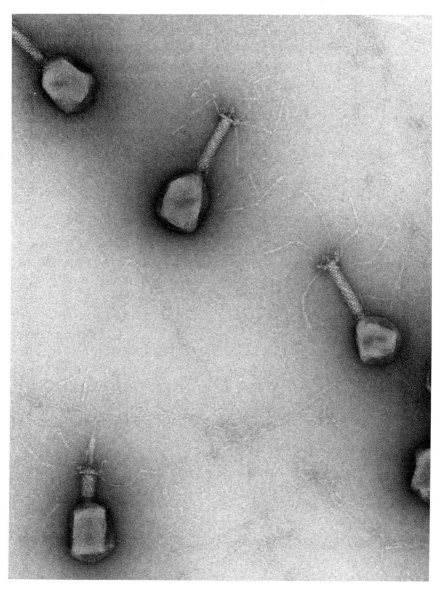

cause symptoms and disease very quickly. Some viruses take months or years to cause sickness. The time it takes for the virus to cause symptoms is called the ***incubation period***. Rabies virus can have an incubation period of 10 days to 1 year and others are much longer. People infected with HIV usually don't show symptoms for 10–11 years.

Bacteria versus Virus Infections

Bacteria are very different from viruses. Bacteria are much larger and more complex and are made of only one cell. Bacteria will grow and multiply if they are given the right temperature, environment, and nutrients (food).

Unlike viruses, bacteria do not need to invade other cells. Usually, they live in harmony with humans, both inside and outside the body. For example, normal bacteria on the skin prevent more dangerous organisms from growing. In our intestines, bacteria aid digestion by breaking down food.

Antibiotics

Sometimes bacteria can get out of control. If bacteria reproduce too rapidly or begin to grow in places they should not be, an infection can occur. Antibiotics are useful tools for controlling bacterial infection (infections caused by bacteria). Antibiotics are chemicals that kill bacteria (Figure 2-6). Overuse or incorrect use of antibiotics can also cause problems.

Both helpful and harmful bacteria are killed by antibiotics. Not finishing a doctor's prescription or taking another person's medication can upset the bodies natural balance of bacteria. This can easily lead to other infections or make the existing infection worse.

Viruses are unaffected by antibiotics. A doctor may prescribe an antibiotic when you catch a flu or cold virus, but this is only to prevent bacterial infections while you are ill.

FIGURE 2–6
A. Antibiotics growing on a laboratory culture dish. *(© Charlotte Raymond, Science Source/Photo Researchers, Inc.)*

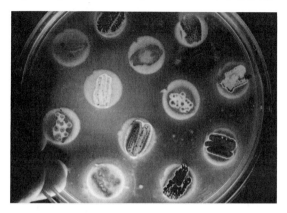

B. Antibiotics inhibiting the growth of bacteria on a culture plate. *(Courtesy of Walters, Estridge, Reynolds.* Basic Medical Laboratory Techniques, *2nd Edition, Delmar Publishers Inc., 1992.)*

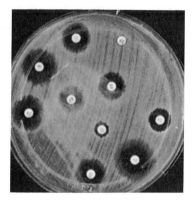

It Is Hard to Be Infected With HIV!

HIV is a very fragile virus that is difficult to spread. Relatively speaking, it's hard to be infected with HIV. Imagine how disastrous it would be if this deadly virus could spread as easily as a cold or flu virus. If this were the case, the world would be faced by an epidemic as serious as the Spanish flu epidemic of 1918. In that great epidemic, as many as 40 million people died in less than two years. In New York City alone, over 5,000 people a day died from this deadly virus.

HIV **cannot** be transmitted by insect bites, sneezing, coughing, hugging, kissing, casual contact, animals, or in food or water. You can share a soda or sandwich with an infected person, even a toothbrush, and not be infected. After many years of study, scientists are convinced that HIV can be spread in only a few ways.

Under normal circumstances only the blood, sperm, and vaginal fluid can transmit HIV to another person. The breast milk of an HIV-positive mother has been shown to sometimes transmit HIV to uninfected babies. HIV is **not** transmitted through feces, nasal secretions, saliva, sweat, tears, urine, or vomit, unless they contain visible blood.[2]

Only certain types of contact with contaminated blood, sperm, or vaginal fluid will cause infection. For example, a person cannot be infected simply by touching HIV-infected blood. Hundreds of health care workers have accidentally touched HIV-infected blood to their skin, eyes, nose, and mouth. Not a single one of these health care workers became infected.

Under normal circumstances, it is difficult for HIV to enter the body and cause infection. HIV-infected blood, sperm, or vaginal fluid can only cause infection in a few ways. They must come in contact with an open sore or wound or the thin delicate tissues called ***mucous membranes***, i.e. the tissue that lines the vagina and inside wall of the anus. (We will discuss contaminated needle sticks later in this chapter.)

Many people have been exposed to HIV-infected blood, sperm, or vaginal fluid and not become infected. A common myth is that having sex with an HIV-infected person always results in infection. This is untrue. Many people have had multiple exposures to HIV and not been infected.

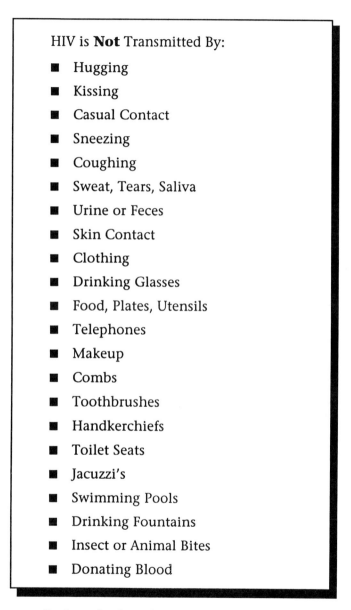

HIV is **Not** Transmitted By:
- Hugging
- Kissing
- Casual Contact
- Sneezing
- Coughing
- Sweat, Tears, Saliva
- Urine or Feces
- Skin Contact
- Clothing
- Drinking Glasses
- Food, Plates, Utensils
- Telephones
- Makeup
- Combs
- Toothbrushes
- Handkerchiefs
- Toilet Seats
- Jacuzzi's
- Swimming Pools
- Drinking Fountains
- Insect or Animal Bites
- Donating Blood

One medical study found only 20% of the females with HIV-infected male partners became infected.[3] This same study also found that it is almost 18 times easier for a man to transmit HIV to a woman than vice versa.

If you know someone who injects drugs, you can help. If you can get the user into a drug counseling center or rehabilitation program, all the better. If not, at least educate the person about HIV and how it spreads. Education is the most important thing in the world. Education can prevent disease, and prevention is always better than any medicine or miracle cure.

The second most risky type of behavior is anal sex. Having unprotected sex with an HIV-infected person does not always spread HIV. However, anal sex greatly increases the risks. During anal sex, tiny tears are made in the inside wall of the anus. HIV is often found in very high amounts in sperm. During anal sex, the virus may enter the blood stream through these small tears. Medical studies show that women are 2–3 times more likely to be infected if they participate in anal sex.[4] Other studies have shown that over 90% of all new infections in gay men are a result of anal sex.[5]

Sexually Transmitted Diseases (STDs)

All anal sex is risky, but certain things can make it more dangerous. If you or your partner has a history of *sexually transmitted diseases (STDs)*, your chances of being infected are increased. Some examples of STDs are:

- chlamydia (cla-**MID**-ee-ah)
- gonorrhea
- herpes
- syphilis
- hepatitis B
- genital warts
- pelvic inflammatory disease (PID)

STDs can also increase the chance of being infected for those who never practice anal sex. Vaginal sex is many times safer than anal sex. However, STDs can increase the chance of passing HIV for both anal and vaginal sex. No one is completely sure of why STDs increase the risks. Many believe it is related to the open sores or damaged skin that frequently appear on the penis or in the vagina. Sores and broken or damaged skin make it much easier for the HIV to enter your body.

After anal sex, the third riskiest type of behavior is having sex with a person who injects drugs. Studies from the first 10 years of the AIDS epidemic have revealed some useful information. Approximately 3% of all people with AIDS became infected because they had sex with a person who injected drugs.

In many Pattern II countries, health care and education are very poor. HIV spread through parts of Africa for many years before it was discovered. Between 60 and 80% of the prostitutes in Pattern II countries are now infected with HIV.[6]

Being sexually involved with a person from a Pattern II country increases your risks. During the first 11 years of the AIDS epidemic 3,630 reported cases of AIDS (5.2% of all cases reported to the CDC) are believed to have been caused by having sex with a person born in a Pattern II country.

Bisexual men rarely transmit HIV to women. Out of the first 174,893 AIDS cases reported only 544 women became infected by having sex with a bisexual male.[7] That is only 0.3% of the total reported cases of AIDS during the first ten years of the epidemic. Lesbians do not transmit HIV between themselves. There has never been a case where a woman infected another woman with HIV.

Blood Transfusions

In recent years, the blood supply in our country has become very safe. Today, HIV is rarely transmitted by blood transfusion. In the first 10 years of the AIDS epidemic, only 3,904 cases (2.2%) were caused by blood transfusions. Government and health officials responded quickly to protect the blood supply through better screening and testing.

Catching HIV from a person who became infected by a blood transfusion is also fairly rare. Of the cases reported in the first 10 years of the epidemic, only 179 people (0.1%) became infected in this way.

AIDS Trends in the United States

Some experts believe that the number of HIV infections in the United States are falling. Others believe they have only stabilized and some categories have not yet peaked. In either case, Figure 2–7 clearly shows that the number of cases is not climbing rapidly, as many Americans fear.

The graph shows a steady increase among heterosexuals. However, the overall numbers of cases reported each year is very small. You can see why the media prefers to report the percentage increase in AIDS cases, instead of actual figures.

From 1991 to 1992 reported AIDS cases among heterosexuals rose from 9,631 to 13,292. It sounds much more frightening to say AIDS cases among heterosexuals rose by over 27.5%. Both are true, but using percentages is obviously deceiving. Who would be frightened to hear that between 1991 and 1992, 3,661 additional heterosexuals in the entire United States population of over 256 million were diagnosed with AIDS? Certainly a 27.5% increase sounds much more alarming.

Trends in the number of reported cases each year provide important information. You must remember that the number of cases this year reflects the number of infections that occurred about 10 years ago. This is because the average time between HIV infection and AIDS is about 10 years.

Statistics show that about mid-1987, fewer numbers of AIDS cases were reported, especially among homosexuals with no history of injecting drugs.[8] Many believe this trend continues. The slowing is attributed to better medicine to

FIGURE 2–7

Four-year trend of AIDS cases reported to the Center for Disease Control.
NOTE: Teen AIDS cases are less than 170 per year.

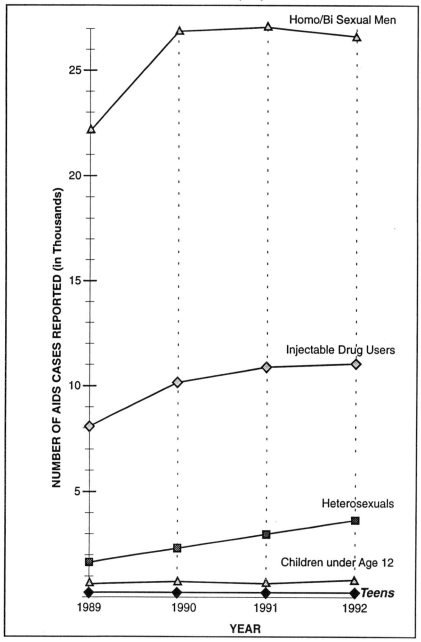

combat AIDS and increased awareness and education in the gay community.

Factors that Increase the Risks

In the United States, people fall under three basic categories:

1. At risk

2. Has sex with an at-risk person

3. Not at risk

Many people who are not at risk (category 3), fear they are at risk (category 1) because they don't understand the real dangers. Certain behaviors or lifestyles are considered riskier than others, just as certain driving habits are more dangerous than others. If you don't participate in the behavior that puts you at risk, you stand a much less chance of being infected. If you also avoid sex with an at-risk person (category 1), your chances of being infected are very, very small—maybe nearly zero!

Controlling the Risks

Let's examine these risks and learn how to avoid them and help stop the spread of HIV and other infectious diseases.

Behavior that places a person at risk is:

- Injecting illegal drugs

- Sharing needles and syringes

- Having anal sex

- Prostitution

- A history of sexually transmitted diseases

- Living or being born in a Pattern II country

Where you live and who you chose to have sex with can increase the risks:

- Living in poor, inner cities
- Sex with people who inject drugs
- Sex with male homosexuals
- Sex with prostitutes
- Sex with people born in Pattern II countries

You can lower your risks to nearly zero if you:

- Avoid at-risk behaviors
- Avoid sex with people who are at risk
- Always use condoms

Smart Sex

Using condoms is smart for many reasons. Remember, sexually transmitted diseases like herpes, syphilis, and gonorrhea haven't gone away. You are far more likely to catch one of these diseases than you are to get AIDS.

In 1991 over half a million people (602,577) in the United States were treated for gonorrhea and another 41,006 for syphilis. About 86% of all STDs occur in people between the ages of 15 and 29.[9] STDs increase your risks of HIV infection and can permanently damage your health. Consider the dangers and be smart—use condoms.

If these diseases aren't reason enough to use condoms, then consider the approximately one million adolescent females who become pregnant each year. Condoms could prevent hundreds of thousands of unwanted babies from being born and many lives from being ruined.

Getting AIDS from Doctors or Dentists

Many people are concerned that their doctor or dentist may infect them with HIV. This is extremely unlikely! These fears come from a poor understanding of HIV and AIDS.

It is highly unlikely that a patient would be infected by a physician, surgeon, or dentist. The chance of being infected by a health care worker has been estimated at 1 in 20 million.[10] A health care worker is far more likely to be infected by a patient. However, even this rarely occurs.

Approximately 1 billion dental procedures are performed each year in the United States.[11] That's about 12 billion procedures between 1981 and 1992. During all of this time, only once has a dentist infected his patients. Obviously the risks are extremely low. In fact, they are nearly zero. You have a much greater chance of being killed in an automobile accident on the way to a doctor or dental appointment. Actually, you are four times more likely to be killed by a bee sting than infected with HIV by a doctor.

Figure 2–8 shows the results of a poll that asked people if they thought certain professionals should be allowed to continue working if they had AIDS. The results of this poll are a reflection of Americans' fear of AIDS. It is silly to think that bus drivers, teachers, or lawyers would spread HIV simply by doing their jobs. To prevent job discrimination, the federal government enacted the ***Americans with Disabilities Act of 1990*** to protect all disabled or handicapped individuals from discrimination in areas of employment, public accommodations, transportation, and telecommunications. This law ensures that no person will be discriminated against because of a physical, mental, or medical disability. People with HIV/AIDS deserve our compassion, not our contempt and prejudice.

Protect Yourself and Clients from All Diseases

Your chances of catching HIV from a client are nearly zero. The same is true of getting HIV from an infected hairdresser, nail technician, esthetician, or other beauty professional. It has never happened and probably never will.

FIGURE 2–8

Percentage of people who believe a person in one of the listed professions should not be allowed to keep working if diagnosed with AIDS. *(Source: AIDS Reference Guide, Dec. 1989, n934, p. 2)*

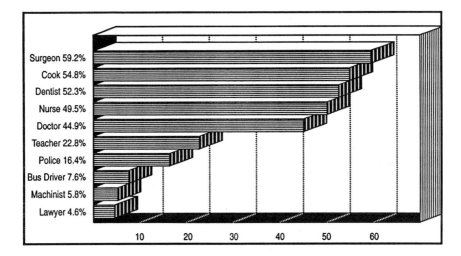

Surgeon 59.2%
Cook 54.8%
Dentist 52.3%
Nurse 49.5%
Doctor 44.9%
Teacher 22.8%
Police 16.4%
Bus Driver 7.6%
Machinist 5.8%
Lawyer 4.6%

10   20   30   40   50   60

Unfortunately, you can bet that if it ever does happen, even once, the media will spring on the story with their fangs bared. Let's hope this never occurs. Under the harsh and often distorted spotlight of the American news media, even one such case would be disastrous to the professional beauty industry.

You must remember that AIDS isn't the only disease in the world. Many other diseases are transmitted far easier. In chapter 6, you will learn that hepatitis is at least 100 times more infectious than HIV. Hepatitis is a much more serious threat in the salon than AIDS.

Cosmetologists, nail technicians, and estheticians are exposed to dozens of people every day. If you are not careful, you could cause your own local epidemic. Many of the same things that don't spread HIV, **do** spread other infectious organisms. In later chapters, you'll learn vital techniques for controlling disease. These techniques (and other information in this book) are important professional tools. Learn them and use them—your clients expect nothing less!

❏ FAST TRACK

1. The human body is a group of many different organs arranged into systems, i.e. the respiratory system and the circulatory system. Many such systems work together to maintain a healthy body.

2. Organs are a group of many smaller cells, i.e. kidney cells and heart cells. Plants are also made of cells that are similar to those in the human body.

3. Cells are the smallest and simplest unit capable of being alive. Cells use nutrients to make substances necessary for life and reproduction.

4. Bacteria are called microorganisms (micro meaning small and organism meaning living creature).

5. Bacteria contain many internal organs for transporting food and waste products, as well as building proteins and other useful substances needed to grow and reproduce.

6. Bacteria use DNA to reproduce in the same way humans do.

7. DNA is a tiny molecule that carries the information needed to reproduce.

8. Amino acids are arranged on the DNA ribbons to spell out a code called the genetic code. The genetic code determines, among other things, whether you will have blue eyes or brown, long legs or short.

9. All living things—trees, insects, rodents, birds, fish— use DNA to reproduce.

10. Viruses are parasites that can only live inside another cell or host cell. Viruses exist in between the world of the living and nonliving. They are too simple to make their own energy, grow, or reproduce.

11. Viruses cause many human illnesses, such as chicken pox, smallpox, influenza (flu), measles, mumps, rubella, rabies, typhoid fever, yellow fever, cold sores, herpes, AIDS, hepatitis, warts, polio, and certain kinds of cancer. At least 30 different viruses can cause the symptoms of a common cold.

12. Viruses must invade or infect other cells. Once the virus infects a host cell, it can grow and reproduce.

13. The time it takes for the virus to cause symptoms is called the incubation period.

14. Antibiotics are used to control infections caused by bacteria, but both helpful and harmful bacteria are killed by antibiotics.

15. Viruses are not affected by antibiotics.

16. HIV is very fragile and difficult to spread.

17. HIV **cannot** be transmitted by insect bites, sneezing, coughing, hugging, kissing, casual contact, animals, or in food or water. You can share a soda or sandwich with an infected person, even a toothbrush, and not be infected.

18. Only blood, sperm, vaginal fluid, and breast milk can transmit HIV to another person.

19. Hundreds of health care workers have accidentally touched HIV-infected blood to their skin, eyes, nose, and mouth without being infected.

20. The surest way to be infected with HIV is by sharing needles or syringes.

21. The spread of HIV among homosexuals is dropping rapidly due to the gay community's organized war of education against AIDS.

22. Anal sex is considered to be the second most likely way to transmit HIV. During anal sex, tiny tears are made in the inside wall of the anus. The virus in the sperm of infected men may enter the bloodstream through these small tears.

23. A history of sexually transmitted diseases (STDs) increases your chances of being infected.

24. Third world or developing countries where HIV spreads mostly through prostitution and male/female sex are called Pattern II countries, i.e. parts of Africa.

25. Bisexual men rarely transmit HIV to women. Only 0.3% of the total reported cases of AIDS during the first 10 years of the epidemic were from sex between bisexual men and women.

26. Today, HIV is rarely transmitted by blood transfusion.

27. Factors that increase your risks of catching HIV are sharing needles and syringes; anal sex; sex with prostitutes; a history of sexually transmitted diseases; living or being born in a developing country; living in poor, inner cities; sex with people who are at risk.

28. You can lower your risk of HIV infection if you avoid at-risk behaviors, avoid sex with people who are at risk, and always use condoms during sex.

29. It has been estimated that the chance of being infected by a health care worker is 1 in 20 million.

30. Over 12 billion dental procedures have been performed between 1981 and 1992 with only one dentist infecting his patients.

31. The Americans with Disabilities Act of 1990 prohibits discrimination against people with HIV/AIDS.

❏ TEST YOUR KNOWLEDGE

Answers are in Appendix B.

1. _____ are the smallest and simplest units capable of being alive.

2. Bacteria are called micro _____.

3. Where do both bacteria and human cells store the genetic code?

4. Viruses are _____ that can only live inside another cell called the ____cell.

5. Which are killed by antibiotics, bacteria or viruses?

6. HIV can only be spread by _____ -to- _____ contact.

7. Name the two most common behaviors that spread HIV.

8. The HIV infection rate among homosexuals is _____, and the rate among people who inject drugs is _____.

9. The chance of being infected with HIV by a health care worker is about 1 in _____.

10. The chance of a salon professional being infected with HIV by a client is nearly _____.

❏ REFERENCE NOTES

1. *AIDS Reference Guide,* (1988, April).

2. *AIDS Reference Guide,* (1988, September).

3. *JAMA, 267* (14), (1992, April 8), p. 1917.

4. Ibid.

5. *JAMA, 264* (2), (1990, July 11), p. 230.

6. Levine, Arnold J. (1992). *Viruses* (p. 142). New York: Scientific American Library.

7. *AIDS Reference Guide,* (1991, June).

8. *JAMA, 262* (11), (1990, March 16), p. 1477.

9. *Morbidity and Mortality Weekly Report (MMWR). 40* (51 & 52), (1992, January 3). Published by *The New England Journal of Medicine.*

10. *JAMA, 267* (10), (1992, March 11), p. 1368.

11. Statistics from the California Dental Association's flyer "AIDS and the Dental Office: What Your Dentist Is Doing to Keep You Safe." California Dental Association, P.O. Box 13749, Sacramento, CA 95853-4749.

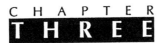

C H A P T E R
THREE

HIV and the Immune System

Each person has command of a great army. This massive fighting force is able to wage a full-scale war upon any foreign aggressor. This army has privates and generals, spies and assassins, sentries and scouts. This army never sleeps. It is constantly prepared to do battle and defend the home front at a moment's notice. This army is inside your body and is called the immune system.

We live in a hostile world, surrounded by invisible invaders such as bacteria, fungi, and viruses. If our bodies did not have some way of defending against attack, we could not live anywhere on Earth.

The immune system gives us *immunity* or protection from disease. This immunity can be natural or acquired. *Natural immunity* is determined genetically. In other words, the genetic code in DNA (see chapter 2) gives us our natural immunity.

How the Immune System Works

Acquired immunity comes from successfully fighting off a disease, like childhood mumps or chicken pox. The other way to acquire an immunity is by being *vaccinated* against a disease.

Vaccines are usually made from bacteria or viruses that have been killed or weakened. For example, when you receive a flu vaccination, the doctor is injecting weakened or destroyed flu viruses into your body. The immune system does not know the virus has been destroyed. It believes the virus is a foreign body or intruder.

The immune system can tell the difference between friends and foes. Viruses and bacteria wear "overcoats" made of protein. Each type of virus or bacteria has a distinctive protein overcoat, much like soldiers from the same country wearing the same uniform. Scientists call these overcoats ***protein envelopes***.

When weakened or destroyed flu viruses are injected into the body, the immune system springs into action. Certain parts of the immune system act as spies. They memorize the uniform (protein overcoat) of the flu virus and send messengers to the generals who organize the attack. The generals send out messengers to alert the immune system army of a possible invasion. They also describe what type of protein overcoat to watch for. The rest of the immune system builds up its defenses and patiently waits for the attack.

Of course, the weakened flu virus is quickly destroyed, but the immune system is ready and stays on the lookout. If the body is later infected by the flu virus, the immune system is ready and waiting. The illness will be milder than if no vaccination had been given. There may be no symptoms at all. As you can see, vaccinations prepare the immune system for future attacks.

Some types of vaccinations produce very strong ***immune responses***. Strong responses can protect the body for many years. Tetanus vaccines, for example, are repeated every 10 years to keep the immune system ready. Measles and mumps vaccines are also long lasting.

Influenza (flu) vaccines are usually required each year mainly because there are many ***strains*** or types of flu viruses. Sometimes, a virus can change or ***mutate***. When a virus mutates, the protein overcoat may also change. If the new protein coat is similar to the old one, the immune system can still recognize it and attack. But many times the immune system is fooled by the new protein overcoat. If you recall from chapter 2, at least 30 different viruses can cause the symptoms of a common cold. These are all **mutations** or slightly altered versions of the same viruses.

Even without a vaccination, the immune system can successfully destroy most viruses. After winning the battle, the immune system remembers the virus's overcoat and stays on the lookout.

Sentries of the Body

What actually remains on the lookout? White blood cells (part of the immune system) produce chemical substances called **antibodies** (anti meaning against and body meaning bacteria, virus, fungus, or other foreign protein). Antibodies are like sentries or guards who watch for the repeat invasions.

Antibodies can stop viruses by sticking to their protein overcoat. Immune system messengers tell the white blood cells about the virus's protein coat. The white blood cells then make antibodies that fit tightly into openings or holes in the virus's overcoat. The antibodies attach the way a key fits into a lock. The shape of the key must match the hole in the lock. Antibodies that match the opening or space in the virus will stick tightly (Figure 3–1 on page 56).

Antibodies in Action

How does this help fight viruses? We learned in chapter 2 that a virus must get inside a host cell before it can reproduce. With an antibody stuck on the overcoat, the virus cannot get inside the host cell. Certain antibodies can tell which host cells contain a virus. These antibodies stick to the outside of the infected host cell and call for help.

FIGURE 3–1

Computer graphic depiction of many antibodies attaching to the outside of a virus particle. *(From: VIRUSES by A.J. Levine. Copyright © 1991 by W.H. Freeman and Company. Reprinted by permission.)*

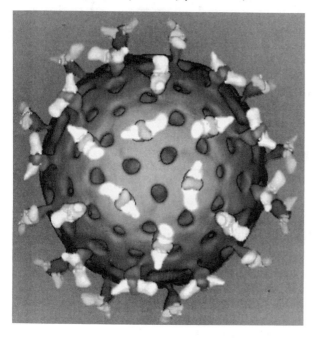

The antibodies send out chemical messages that attract other immune cells called **killer T cells.** These cells are like soldiers. They respond to the antibodies call for help. Killer T cells bore a hole in the infected cell and inject substances that destroy the virus.

Other types of cells roam the body like assassins, looking for invaders. Some look for antibodies attached to the overcoats of the intruders. Others automatically attack all foreign bodies.

Some types of cells act like instigators to get the other cells "fired up" for battle. These cells are called **helper T cells** or CD4 cells. (CD4 is actually a small section of the cell that acts as a doorway for HIV.) These cells are **extremely**

important because they make killer cells more effective. Without helper T cells, the army would have no direction or focus. It would be like a professional football team without a coach. In some ways, helper T cells are the most important cells in the immune system.

The immune system has many types of cells each performing an important job. You do not need to memorize all the different cells' names. What is important is to understand the way the immune system works. It is a team effort, with many players. It is a complex and efficient system, but sometimes things can go wrong.

When Things Go Wrong

Even the immune system makes bloopers. For instance, the body will sometimes reject a heart transplant. This is the immune system's fault. Transplants often fool parts of the immune system into attacking friendly immune cells, much like an army fighting against its own troops. The resulting battle can lay waste to the entire immune system.

AIDS is another example of what can happen when things go wrong. The AIDS virus causes the immune system to break down. What better way to win a war than to paralyze the defender's army? This is how HIV causes AIDS.

Before we continue, let's review what we have learned about HIV and other viruses.

- Viruses are parasites that can only live inside another cell or host cell.

- Viruses exist in between the world of the living and nonliving. They are too simple to make their own energy, grow, or reproduce.

- Viruses cause illness in humans, animals, and plants.

- Viruses must invade or infect other cells. Once the virus infects a host cell, it can grow and reproduce.

- Viruses prefer to use certain types of cells as hosts.

- The time it takes for the virus to cause symptoms is called the incubation period.

- Viruses are not affected by antibiotics.

- HIV (human immunodeficiency virus) is fragile and difficult to spread.

- HIV **cannot** be transmitted by insect bites, sneezing, coughing, hugging, kissing, casual contact, animals, or in food or water.

- HIV can only be spread through infected blood, semen, vaginal fluid, and breast milk.

HIV Versus the Immune System

How does HIV destroy the immune system? What happens once the virus enters the body? Scientists do not have all the details yet, but much is known about HIV and how it attacks.

Once HIV gets into the bloodstream, like many viruses it seeks out its favorite cell to act as a host. If that type of cell was a skin cell or some other tissue of lesser importance, HIV would never have become the most dreaded virus of our time. Unfortunately, HIV likes to use immune system cells as hosts. Even worse, HIV infects helper T cells, one of the most important parts of the immune system.

If you recall, helper T cells are the coaches for the immune system. Without helper T cells, the immune system loses much of its focus and purpose. HIV recognizes a helper T cell by its protein coat (the same trick that immune cells use to recognize invaders).

Part of HIV fits into a space on the overcoat of the helper T cell (like a lock and key). Once it attaches itself to the helper T cell, it bores a hole and enters the host cell (Figure 3–2). The virus can now do one of many things. It may sit quietly

FIGURE 3–2
HIV attaching to a helper T cell. *(From: VIRUSES by A.J. Levine. Copyright © 1991 by W.H. Freeman and Company. Reprinted by permission.)*

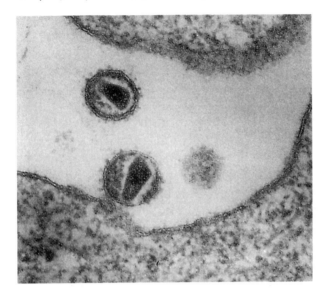

inside the cell for many years without causing illness or symptoms. (If you recall, this is called the incubation period.) The virus can also begin to reproduce, making hundreds of copies of itself.

Quiet—But Not Asleep

In 1993, scientists made an important discovery. Although HIV does not produce symptoms for many years, it is not inactive. New findings show that HIV becomes trapped by special glands called **lymph nodes**.

These small, bean-shaped structures are part of the immune system. They are designed to filter the blood and destroy foreign substances, such as bacteria. They are found in the throat, armpits, inside the elbow or knee, behind the ear, in the groin area, and other places.

The lymph glands serve as a "hideout" for HIV. From there, the virus can reproduce and quietly begin to infiltrate the immune system's defenses. During the early stages of infection, the lymph glands hold about 100 billion HIV-infected helper T cells. As many as 1 billion of these are actively reproducing.[1]

HIV—The Retrovirus

There are many groups or families of viruses. HIV belongs to the family of *retroviruses* (retro meaning backward). Until the late seventies scientists did not study the retroviruses because they did not believe retroviruses caused human disease. But in 1977, researchers began to believe that a certain type of leukemia (ATL or adult T-cell leukemia) was caused by a retrovirus. Soon, scientists all around the world were studying retroviruses. One year before the AIDS epidemic was discovered, scientists proved that retroviruses could cause a type of leukemia.

HIV and other retroviruses are unique in the way they reproduce. Remember from the last chapter:

1. Viruses are too simple to reproduce on their own.

2. DNA carries the genetic code that tells cells how to reproduce.

Amazingly, HIV has no DNA! Then how does it reproduce? It makes the host cell's genetic machinery work backwards. While this is happening, HIV changes the DNA code of the host cell. This is what makes HIV a retro, or "backward" virus.

Changing the DNA code forces the helper T cell to make more HIV, instead of more helper T cells. This is sort of like making a cat have puppies. Once the host cell makes hundreds of copies of the HIV, it bursts open, spreading the new HIVs. They, in turn, infect hundreds of other helper T cells and repeat the cycle.

This is why HIV infections are so deadly. In a sense, HIV turns the helper T cells into double-agents. They no longer can "coach" the immune system team and they are forced to make more HIV! The spreading viruses infect more and more helper T cells until there are very few healthy ones left. Without them, the body can't defend itself from **any** attacker.

Many types of bacteria and viruses live inside the body. The immune system acts like a prison guard keeping them strictly under control. Without helper T cells, they are suddenly free to grow out of control (Figure 3-3).

Of course, the immune system does not just give up and quit. Quite the contrary. The immune system fights back for as long as it is able. The white blood cells make the antibodies, which stick to HIV overcoats and the outside of infected host cells. The killer cells then zoom in and destroy the virus and infected cells. But as more and more helper T cells become infected, the immune system can't keep up with the ever-increasing numbers of new HIVs. Soon there are too many to destroy.

FIGURE 3-3

New copies of HIV cells budding from the surface of an infected helper T cell. *(From: VIRUSES by A.J. Levine. Copyright © 1991 by W.H. Freeman and Company. Reprinted by permission.)*

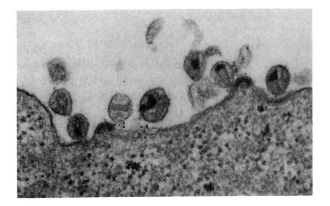

All of this confusion and uproar in the immune system allows all types of infections and cancers to grow. This is AIDS! HIV destroys the immune system so that it cannot fight off disease. If an AIDS victim catches the flu, it could be fatal.

When Does a Person Have AIDS?

The answer to this question has changed four times since the beginning of the AIDS epidemic. The latest change was in January 1993. The answer is surprising. You don't have AIDS until the government says you do. The Center for Disease Control (CDC), an agency of the federal government, decides how AIDS is to be defined.

Defining AIDS is actually more difficult than you might imagine. The same diseases that kill people without AIDS kill people because of AIDS. In other words, simply having an AIDS-related disease doesn't mean you're infected with HIV or have AIDS.

At the beginning of the epidemic, no one knew the cause of AIDS. HIV had not been discovered. Many disorders, besides AIDS, cause rapid weight loss and weakness. What if a patient developed cancer? How could doctors know if it was because of AIDS?

HIV Testing

Scientists have now discovered a way to determine if a person is infected with HIV. They can test for the antibodies the immune system makes to fight HIV. The immune system would not make these disease-fighting antibodies unless HIV was present.

The most widely used test is the **EIA** (*enzyme immunoassay* [i-myoo-no-**AS**-say]). In infected persons, the clear liquid portion of blood (serum) contains HIV antibodies. If a person tests positive for HIV antibodies, another test is performed to verify the results. The second test is called the ***Western blot test*** (Figure 3–4). The Western blot test also tests for HIV antibodies in blood serum, but is slightly more reliable. Since the EIA test is less expensive and faster, it is used as a screening test and the Western blot test confirms positive results. The EIA is 99.75% accurate, and the Western blot test is 99.99% accurate.[2]

Occasionally, a person not infected with HIV may test positive. However, as health agencies are extremely careful to verify all positive results, this rarely occurs. It is equally unlikely that a person will test negative when they are actually infected with HIV. This can occur if a person is tested shortly after being infected.

FIGURE 3–4

Immunodetection of HIV-1 using the ELISAmate Western Blot HRP System (left) and AP System (right). *(Photo courtesy of Kirkegaard & Perry Laboratories, Inc., Gaithersburg, Maryland.)*

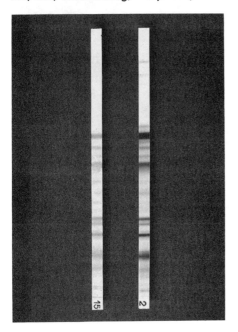

Doctors use another test to determine how serious an HIV infection has become. From a blood sample, doctors can measure how many helper T cells the infected person has. The Center for Disease Control uses the number of CD4 (same as helper T cells) cells to determine if a person has developed AIDS. When a person's helper T cells fall below a certain level, the immune system can no longer function.[a]

AIDS is not the only factor that decreases levels of helper T cells. In 1992, it was learned that between 45 and 50 people showed symptoms of AIDS-like illness, but were not HIV positive. They also had helper T cell levels typical of people with AIDS. After months of study, researchers determined that these people had an extremely rare disorder completely unrelated to HIV infections.[3]

HIV-2 Testing

There are two types of viruses known to cause AIDS, HIV-1 and HIV-2. The media caused an uproar when it was discovered that the EIA screening test could not tell if blood was infected with HIV-2.

Headlines screamed about our "questionable" and "unsafe" blood supply. It was suggested that many people may have received transfusions from blood infected with the invisible HIV-2 virus. What the media failed to mention is that only 32 U.S. residents have been discovered to carry HIV-2. The truth is, HIV-2 is not (and never was) a threat to our blood supply. The EIA test now was modified to test for HIV-1 and HIV-2 and the media turned its attention elsewhere.

Window Phase and Mandatory Testing

There is a short period called a **window phase** that immediately follows infection. During the window phase, an infected person may actually test negative, even though

---

a. The CDC's 1992 definition of AIDS is a CD4 count below 200 cells/microliter of blood. Normally, adults have about 800–1200 CD4 cells/microliter of blood.

they are positive. The window phase lasts between three and six months after infection.

Some fear that the window phase makes HIV more easily spread. However, studies indicate that there is only a small probablility that a person infected with HIV will escape detection simply because of the window phase.[4]

People sometimes wonder why there is no mandatory nationwide HIV testing. Unfortunately, the cost would be staggering and the benefits questionable. The most important people to test are also the ones who would be least likely to be tested. Poor, inner-city dwellers, transients, prostitutes, and injected drug users are difficult enough to count each census year. Testing all high-risk people would be practically impossible. Besides, testing alone does not prevent the spread of HIV; education and awareness is the answer.

In a Nutshell

HIV is a simple virus. It is not like a horror film monster, taking pleasure in destroying everything it sees. What makes HIV dangerous is that it prefers to live and reproduce in immune system cells. But, something else makes HIV even more dangerous: ignorance and fear.

Humans usually fear what they do not understand. Only knowledge can conquer that fear. Scientists and doctors are doing all they can to understand HIV and how to control it. We need to do the same. With understanding, knowledge, and truth, we can overcome irrational fears and prejudice.

❏ FAST TRACK

1. The immune system gives us immunity or protection from disease.

2. Natural immunity is determined genetically by the genetic code in DNA.

3. Vaccines are usually made from bacteria or viruses that have been killed or weakened.

4. Each type of virus or bacteria has a distinctive protein overcoat.

5. Viruses can change or mutate.

6. White blood cells produce chemical substances called antibodies that are like sentries or guards, watching for the return of the invaders.

7. One way antibodies can stop viruses is by sticking to their protein overcoat.

8. The antibodies can send out chemical messages to attract killer T cells.

9. Helper T cells are the coaches of the immune system; they make killer T cells work more effectively.

10. The HIV virus causes the immune system to break down.

11. HIV uses helper T cells as host cells.

12. HIV recognizes helper T cells by their protein coat.

13. HIV belongs to the family of retroviruses (retro meaning backward).

14. Since HIV has no DNA, it tricks helper T cells into making more copies of HIV. Once the helper T cell has made hundreds of copies of the HIV, it bursts open and spreads the new HIVs, which infect hundreds of other helper T cells.

15. The HIV tests look for antibodies the immune system makes to fight HIV.

16. The most widely used HIV test is the EIA.

17. A positive EIA test is confirmed with a Western blot test.

18. In the short window phase, a person may test HIV negative, even if they are positive.

19. People infected with HIV can spread the virus—even if they have no symptoms.

❏ TEST YOUR KNOWLEDGE

Answers are in Appendix B.

1. Name the system that protects our bodies from infection and many diseases.

2. How does the immune system recognize most invaders?

3. Viruses can change or _____.

4. _____ cells act as coaches for the immune system and host cells for HIV.

5. Why can't HIV reproduce by itself? What does it need?

6. _____ are usually made from bacteria or viruses that have been killed or weakened.

7. The most widely used test for HIV is _____.

8. In infected persons, HIV antibodies are found in the _____.

9. Another test called the _____ is performed to verify HIV-positive results.

10. To be sure an HIV test is negative, it must be taken after the end of the _____ phase that lasts from ___ to ___ months.

❏ REFERENCE NOTES

1. Pennisi, E. (1993, March). HIV: Out of sight but not inactive. *Science News, 143* (13), p. 196.

2. *AIDS Reference Guide, sec. 907,* (1988, April), p. 12.

3. Fackelmann, K. A. (1993, February). Immune system remains mysterious. *Science News, 143* (8), p. 119.

4. *AIDS Reference Guide,* (1988, April).

CHAPTER FOUR

AIDS and ARC

AIDS has the distinction of being the first major human epidemic to be fought with modern advertising techniques. Catchy phrases like "AIDS doesn't discriminate" and "Anyone can get AIDS" have become part of our everyday conversations. Although there is some truth to these statements, they are oversimplifications.

Does AIDS really not discriminate? Does everyone really have the same likelihood of being infected with HIV? Let's explore the answers to these and other questions.

We have learned why people get AIDS, now let's look at who gets this disease and learn about the symptoms.

Who Gets AIDS?

There is only one way to get AIDS. You must be infected with the virus known as HIV. HIV does not strike at random. Researchers have discovered certain patterns of behavior that cause HIV to be transmitted. Research has also shown that the risk of catching HIV depends greatly upon where you live. (Both of these factors were discussed in previous chapters.)

Of course, anyone can become infected with HIV. Anyone can be attacked by a shark or struck by lightning. However, if you have only been swimming in the ocean once or twice and you never go out in a thunderstorm, the chances are very small that either will happen to you. On the other hand, if you like to spearfish off the Great Barrier Reef or play golf on stormy days, your chances are increased enormously!

AIDS is not just for homosexuals, prostitutes, and drug users. Anyone can get AIDS, but you can easily lower your risk to nearly zero. Fortunately, it is hard to become infected with HIV. Many people have been repeatedly exposed without being infected. This, however, does not mean you should not take precautions to protect yourself. Let's review what we learned in chapter 2.

HIV Risk-Increasing Behavior

Ways to increase your risks:

- Injecting illegal drugs
- Sharing needles and syringes
- Having anal sex
- Prostitution
- A history of sexually transmitted diseases
- Living in poor, inner cities
- Living or being born in a Pattern II country, i.e. Central Africa or Haiti
- Sex with people born in Pattern II countries
- Sex with people who inject illegal drugs
- Sex with male homosexuals
- Sex with prostitutes

You can lower your risks to nearly **zero** if you:

- Avoid at-risk behaviors
- Avoid sex with people who are at risk
- Always use condoms

Signs and Symptoms of AIDS and ARC

The symptoms of AIDS usually occur many years after infection. On the average, about 10 to 11 years will pass before infected individuals begin to show symptoms. (Occasionally a person may develop AIDS symptoms only a few months after infection, but these are rare exceptions.) It is important to remember that people who carry HIV can spread the virus—even if they have no symptoms.

First Signs

Generally the first symptoms of HIV infection occur about three months after infection. Flulike symptoms with diarrhea, nausea, aching muscles, and a tired feeling usually occur and quickly go away. Although infected with HIV, the person does not have AIDS. Many years may go by before AIDS symptoms appear.

Symptoms of ARC

When the virus begins to rapidly grow and spread, symptoms follow quickly. The infected person begins to develop a general feeling of sickness, called **malaise**. The flulike symptoms also return along with weight loss, night sweats, and fever. At this point, the person has developed **ARC** or **AIDS-related complex**.[a] ARC can last for a few weeks or a few months. The symptoms worsen and progress into other, more serious health problems. When this happens the person has left the ARC stage and developed AIDS.

ARC is a serious health threat, even before it becomes AIDS. It is possible to die from ARC complications before the infection reaches the AIDS stage. It is important that HIV-positive people receive early medical care and appropriate treatment before they develop AIDS. Proper medical care can help people stay healthy for much longer.

---

a. Sometimes called "pre-AIDS"

As the HIV infection spreads, the immune system begins to rapidly break down. The body can no longer protect itself. Bacteria, fungi, or viruses take advantage of the opportunity to infect the body. These are called ***opportunistic infections.***

Besides the symptoms already described, AIDS can cause ***wasting syndrome*** or rapid, uncontrolled weight loss. In Africa, AIDS is called "the thins," because of the great weight loss it causes. Of course, many other things can cause weight loss. One symptom does not mean a person has AIDS. However, rapid weight loss for any reason is a matter for concern and a doctor should be consulted.

The small, bean-shaped ***lymph glands*** (also called lymph nodes) designed to filter the blood may also be affected. These glands are found in the throat, armpits, inside the elbow or knee, behind the ear, in the groin area and other places. Many things, including AIDS, can cause these glands to swell. When this happens they form noticeable lumps below the skin where the gland lies.

Skin sores develop early in most AIDS victims. Usually, these sores occur around the mouth, genitals, anus, and, less commonly, the back and chest. These sores rarely heal and usually worsen with time. ***Herpes simplex*** (herpes) and ***herpes zoster*** (shingles) are common examples. These skin diseases and others are common in AIDS.

Extreme caution must be taken with any skin sore, especially if it is open or raw. Both herpes and shingles can be spread by touching the sore or oozing fluid. This is why it is important that you **never** perform any type of service on clients with skin sores or lesions. Most states have specific rules that require practitioners to send all clients with open sores to doctors. To protect yourself and other clients, insist that a client get a written letter from a qualified medical doctor stating that the sores are not contagious. Although it is highly unlikely, HIV may be transmitted from these open sores.[b]

---

b. This has never occurred in a salon, but the remote possibility exists.

Lung problems are a dangerous symptom of AIDS. Difficulty breathing and constant hacking or coughing often develop. About 16% of the AIDS victims develop a rare type of pneumonia called PCP (***pneumocystis carinii*** [nu-mah-**SIS**-tis kah-**RYE**-nee-ee] pneumonia). Since so many AIDS patients get this usually rare disease, PCP (and other diseases) are called ***AIDS indicators.***

AIDS Indicators

Several diseases are so common among those with AIDS they have become indicators of the syndrome.[1] About 27% develop one or more AIDS-indicator diseases. Kaposi's sarcoma (KS) was a rare disease before the AIDS epidemic. People with AIDS are 20,000 times more likely to develop this disease than those without AIDS.[2] KS is a soft, purplish, raised growth or lesion that spreads from the feet to other parts of the body.

Another AIDS-indicator disease is mouth and throat fungus. Mouth fungus is generally called ***thrush*** (***esophageal candidiasis*** [i-sah-fah-**JEE**-al kan-dah-**DYE**-ah-sis] or ***Candida albicans***). Thrush is a whitish-grey fungus that grows in the mouths of 34% of the people with AIDS. Less often, a similar fungus occurs in the throat.

Mouth ulcers and sores may develop as well. AIDS makes it difficult for sores to heal and can cause abnormal bleeding of the gums and nose.

Many other diseases can occur as well. In Africa, tuberculosis kills most AIDS victims, but this disease occurs in only 3% of the cases in the United States. HIV can also infect brain cells, causing depression, slowed motion and speech, forgetfulness, and confusion. The eyes of about 20% of AIDS victims are infected with another virus called ***cytomegalovirus*** (sye-tah-me-gah-lo-**VYE**-rus) (CMV) that can lead to blindness.

Progression of AIDS

Eventually, the immune system can no longer protect a person with AIDS. Many diseases afflict those with AIDS and one or more of them eventually causes death. However, better treatments and improved medications have dramatically increased the length and quality of life for those suffering from AIDS. Continued breakthroughs should make even greater improvements for the unfortunate victims.

The Four Categories of HIV Infection

People who have been infected with HIV do not necessarily develop AIDS. Many HIV-positive individuals may never get AIDS. However, it is important to remember that anyone who is HIV positive can spread the virus to another person.

HIV-positive people fall into four general categories:

1. Those who have been infected with the virus but have no symptoms.

2. Those who have the warning symptoms of ARC, including swollen lymph glands, malaise, night sweats, fever, and diarrhea.

3. Those who have developed opportunistic diseases, but are not in need of hospitalization.

4. Those with multiple infections or diseases that may require extended hospitalization. This stage is also called **full-blown AIDS.**

People in the first three categories can usually continue to work and lead productive lives. Sadly, many are shunned or discriminated against out of simple fear and ignorance.

The Rights of People with AIDS

We must never forget that AIDS victims are people, just like us—except they are ill. They have friends and families, mothers and fathers, but more importantly, they (like you) have civil rights protected by the U.S. Constitution. Many federal and state regulations protect HIV-positive people from discrimination. Discriminating against an HIV-infected person is no different than discrimination based on race or sex. How a person became ill is of little importance. What matters is that the person be treated with the respect and dignity that all people deserve.

The Americans with Disabilities Act of 1990 protects all disabled or handicapped individuals from discrimination in areas of employment, public accommodations, transportation, and telecommunications. Businesses with more than 14 employees cannot refuse to hire people because they are handicapped, even if they are HIV positive. Neither can employees be fired because they are infected with HIV or physically handicapped, as long as they can reasonably perform their work.

Federal law also prohibits any salon employee from refusing service to an individual who is physically handicapped or infected with HIV. The obvious exception is a client with open sores or lesions that may be infectious. In this case, the practitioner is required to refer the client to a physician to determine if there is a risk of transmitting disease. Should a qualified medical doctor determine there is no risk, salon employees are bound by federal law to provide any service regularly offered to other clients.

As mentioned before, no salon professional has ever been infected with HIV by a client in the workplace. You will be protected if you follow the universal sanitation and disinfection procedures described in chapter 7.

Your Moral Responsibilities

Discrimination in any form is ugly and wasteful. When you become a provider of a public service, you must accept many responsibilities. You have an obligation to protect yourself and your clients from harm and a legal obligation to provide equal services to all patrons. You also have a moral obligation to treat each client with respect and consideration. The facts are, as a salon professional, you have little to fear from HIV-positive clients.

Putting the Pieces Together

AIDS is a syndrome—a group of signs and symptoms that together indicate a disease. If clients have one or more of the symptoms listed in this chapter, it does not mean they have AIDS.

Remember, unless you are in one of the listed high-risk groups, your chance of being infected with HIV is almost zero. Even if your client does have AIDS, the chance of you being infected while performing routine services is virtually nonexistent. During the first 11 years of the AIDS epidemic, no salon employee has been infected by an HIV-positive client.

In the following chapters, you will learn everything you need to know to protect yourself and clients from **all** infectious diseases. AIDS has received most of the public's attention, but there are other diseases. Many lesser-known diseases are far more likely to visit your salon.

Remember, we live in a hostile environment of invisible, microscopic invaders. Your clients and family expect you to use your knowledge and training to control diseases, not spread them.

❏ FAST TRACK

1. On the average, the symptoms of AIDS usually occur 10–11 years after infection has occurred.

2. ARC stands for AIDS-related complex.

3. Symptoms of ARC are usually flulike with diarrhea, nausea, fever, aching muscles, and a tired feeling that does not go away.

4. The infected person begins to develop a general feeling of sickness, called malaise.

5. It is possible to die from ARC before the infection reaches the AIDS stage.

6. The first flulike symptoms of HIV infection usually occur about three months after infection and quickly go away.

7. Opportunistic infections occur when bacteria, fungi, or viruses take advantage of the weakened immune system and cause disease.

8. AIDS can cause wasting syndrome, or rapid, uncontrolled weight loss.

9. Lymph glands are small, bean-shaped structures designed to filter out and destroy foreign substances such as bacteria. In AIDS, lymph glands can swell to form noticeable lumps.

10. Nonhealing, infectious (and noninfectious) skin sores occur early in AIDS. Herpes simplex (herpes) and herpes zoster (shingles) are common examples.

11. Both herpes and shingles can be spread my touch.

12. **Never** perform any type of service on clients with open sores or lesions.

13. AIDS-indicator diseases include pneumonia (PCP), Kaposi's sarcoma, and thrush. Mouth ulcers and sores, tuberculosis, brain disease, and eye infections also occur.

14. AIDS is a syndrome—a group of signs and symptoms that together indicate a disease.

15. The Americans with Disabilities Act of 1990 protects all disabled or handicapped individuals from discrimination in areas of employment, public accommodations, transportation, and telecommunications.

16. Businesses with more than 14 employees cannot refuse to hire people because they are handicapped, even if they are HIV positive. Neither can employees be fired because they are infected with HIV or physically handicapped, as long as they can reasonably perform their work.

17. Federal law also prohibits any salon employee from refusing service to an individual who is physically handicapped or infected with HIV.

18. No salon professional has ever been infected with HIV by a client in the workplace.

19. AIDS has received most of the public's attention, but there are other, lesser-known diseases that are far more likely to visit your salon.

20. Your clients and family expect you to use your knowledge and training to control diseases, not spread them.

❏ TEST YOUR KNOWLEDGE

Answers are in Appendix B.

1. Name the system that protects our bodies from infection and many diseases.

2. _____ infections occur when bacteria, fungi, or viruses take advantage of the weakened immune system and cause disease.

3. _____ _____ are small, bean-shaped structures designed to filter out and destroy foreign substances such as bacteria found in the blood.

4. Give an example of an AIDS-indicator disease.

5. AIDS is a _____—a group of signs and symptoms that together indicate a disease.

6. True or False

Many diseases, besides HIV, are far more likely to be transmitted in the salon.

7. Do all HIV-positive people get AIDS?

8. Can you refuse to provide certain services to a client simply because they are HIV positive?

9. Can you make HIV-positive people sit in another room, away from other clients, to receive services?

❏ REFERENCE NOTES

1. *JAMA, 267* (13), (1992, April 1), p. 1798.

2. *JAMA, 265* (23), (1991, June 19), p. 3111.

F I V E

Advances Against AIDS

People tend to concentrate on the negative things about the epidemic—what we don't know ... but, on the positive side, there has been tremendous advances in knowledge in the past few years.

R. Wykoff, M.D., Director
Food and Drug Administration
Office of AIDS Coordination

Much has been learned about HIV and AIDS. Never before in history have so many dedicated women and men of science worked toward fighting a single virus.

Researchers not only are learning about HIV, but are discovering things that will ultimately lead to the cure of all diseases caused by viruses. In our lifetime, we will witness a knowledge explosion in the field of medicine. Much of this information will improve the health and quality of life for everyone around the world.

Latest Drugs and Treatments

The Food and Drug Administration (FDA) is responsible for approving all new drugs in the United States. A number of important drugs have been approved to combat HIV. Unfortunately, none of them are a cure for AIDS. Still, they are important first steps and will lead to an eventual cure or vaccine.

Retrovir (also called ***Zidovudine*** or ***AZT***) prevents HIV from reproducing. Retrovir slows down the onset of AIDS and ARC. The drug stops helper T cells from making copies of the invading virus. Unfortunately, Retrovir is so toxic to the bone marrow that nearly one third of all people cannot take the drug. Most can only take the drug for a limited time before the side effects make them discontinue use.

Procrit (also called ***Erythropoietin***) lessens the negative side effects and toxicity of Retrovir (AZT). It lowers the toxic effects on the bone marrow and prevents anemia.[a] This useful drug allows people to take Retrovir longer.

Videx (also called ***didanosine*** or ***ddI***) helps the immune system increase the number of helper T cells (CD4 cells) in people who cannot tolerate Retrovir. It works in the same way as Retrovir, blocking reproduction of HIV.

NebuPent or ***Pentam*** (also called ***pentamidine***) both prevent one of the most common causes of death in people with advanced AIDS, a rare form of pneumonia called PCP. These drugs have been extremely successful in preventing this often fatal lung infection.

Cytovene (also called ***Ganciclovir***) treats a common type of eye infection found in those suffering from AIDS.[b] Left untreated, the infection often leads to blindness. Nearly 20% of the people with AIDS develop serious eye infections.

Foscavir (also called ***Foscarnet***) treats the same eye infection mentioned above. Neither Cytovene nor Foscavir are cures; they merely prevent the serious infections and blindness and help to eliminate symptoms. Recent studies have shown Foscavir to be significantly more effective than Cytovene;[1] however it is more toxic to the kidneys.

---

a. A blood disorder caused by too few red blood cells and thus a lower oxygen-carrying ability.
b. The eye infection is called cytomegalovirus, a type of herpes virus that infects the eye.

Roferon-A or **Intron-A** (also called **alpha-interferon**) is used to treat Kaposi's sarcoma, a rare skin cancer found most commonly on male homosexuals with AIDS.

Diflucan (also called **Fluconazole**) treats both thrush, a fungal infection of the mouth, and cryptococcal (krip-toe-**KAH**-kahl) meningitis, a serious bacterial infection of the brain.

About 400 new drugs are currently being tested by the FDA for safety and effectiveness. In order to speed useful drugs to those in need, they have streamlined the new drug approval process. This faster drug approval is due mostly to pressure from AIDS activist groups and doctors who successfully convinced the FDA to shorten the testing on promising AIDS-related drugs.

New Drugs—Why Are They so Hard to Find?

Until 1983, little was known about viruses and nothing was known about HIV. Researchers have discovered much in a very short period of time, despite the enormous challenge they face.

The gay community was the first group hit by HIV and AIDS. They responded rapidly. In the early years of the epidemic hundreds of infected people allowed themselves to be interviewed and many volunteered to participate in experimental studies. Even today, most human volunteers are from the gay community. Uninfected gays have also volunteered to test new vaccines. One man even donated his lymph glands to help in an important research project. Many others have given their lives.

Hope for a Vaccine

Experts agree, the easiest way to stop the spread of HIV is with a safe and effective vaccine that would prevent the spread of HIV to uninfected people.[c] At least eight vaccines are currently being studied in limited human testing. Researchers are looking for a vaccine that will cause the immune system to produce massive amounts of antibodies to fight HIV.

In the past, vaccines have been an extremely effective way of controlling deadly viruses. The smallpox virus was completely eliminated thanks to a worldwide vaccination program. Polio (poliomyelitis) is another vaccine success story. Polio has been around for at least 5,000 years, possibly longer. Before a polio vaccine was discovered in the early fifties, 21,000 cases occurred each year in the United States. These two diseases alone killed or crippled hundreds of millions of people before they were finally stopped by scientific research.

A number of promising HIV vaccines have been found. Many of these are being tested in humans, even though the animal trials have not been completed. Only time will tell if they are effective.

Why Is It So Difficult to Find a Cure?

It is no easy task to develop a cure for viruses. Since their discovery 100 years ago, they have eluded and outwitted the finest scientific minds the world has ever seen. However, the more we learn about them, the more certain it is that we will learn to control them.

The first thing researchers must prove is that a potential vaccine is safe and will not cause dangerous side effects. Second, they must prove it completely protects the vaccinated person. There are hundreds of drugs that slow HIV's growth or kill it completely in the test tube. Most drugs

---

c. It is possible that a vaccine could work in people already infected with HIV. For example, the rabies vaccine works even after infection has occurred.

never make it past the test tube because they prove to be unsafe or not very effective in humans.

Although HIV prefers to infect helper T cells, other types of cells are also infected. This poses a big problem for researchers. Drugs that could wipe out HIV from all the different types of infected tissue would probably do great damage to healthy tissues, too. Another problem is that HIV is constantly mutating (changing slightly). A successful drug must stop all strains or types of HIV and be free from serious side effects.

Discovering one vaccine may not be enough. Most scientists agree that a mixture or "cocktail" of different drugs may prove to be the most effective. To make matters more confusing, three different vaccines will probably be needed.[2]

1. To prevent infection in people who are not infected with HIV.

2. To slow or stop the infection in people who are HIV positive or have AIDS.

3. To prevent pregnant HIV carriers from infecting their unborn children at birth.

The expense of bringing any new drug to the marketplace is staggering. It can cost tens of millions of dollars to get approval for a single prescription drug. Many years of research and millions of dollars can be spent on a promising HIV/AIDS drug only to find it does not work very well or makes patients too sick.

The Dark Side of the AIDS Epidemic

Sadly, some people have found a way to make money from phony and "bootlegged" AIDS drugs. Many underground AIDS groups are supplying HIV-infected people with home-made, poor quality versions of prescription HIV/AIDS drugs. Some of these prescription drugs are experimental and still undergoing testing. Their safety and effectiveness are unknown.

Unscrupulous individuals are also selling untested, phony "treatments and cures." Several deaths have resulted from these underground medicines.

Why Must We Use Animals for Testing?

Scientists are not born in test tubes, given white coats, and raised in laboratories. They are people, women and men, just like you. They have children, go on picnics, and, yes, they love animals, too. Scientists have pets—dogs and cats, birds and fish—the same as anyone else. Have you ever stopped to wonder why scientists insist on using animals in their research? The answer is clear; because they must!

Although not the most pleasant topic, animal testing must be discussed. Like it or not, your health and the health of your family depends upon animal testing. Everyone born or raised in the United States has benefited in some way from animal research. In fact, this holds true for much of the civilized world. Many adults and children owe their lives to animal research.

All new medicines and breakthrough medical procedures must first be tested to determine if they are safe. Who would want to give a new, untested medicine for cholera to an infant already weakened by this deadly ailment?

Many strongly believe that animal testing is wrong. Strangely, many of these are the same people who scream that not enough is being done to find a cure for AIDS. They do not realize; it can't be both ways. A vaccine or cure will never be discovered without the help of animals.

Americans frequently do not get the whole story from the media. What we hear is usually distorted or incomplete. This lack of balanced information causes people to base their opinions largely on emotion, instead of the truth. We often make judgments about extremely important matters without knowing the facts. How we feel has become more important than right or wrong. Being responsible members of society, we should get **all the facts** before making hasty judgments.

It is important to know what we believe in and why. Instead, we often believe in things that "sound" right. This is a dangerous habit. We must look at the facts, both past and present. Hopefully, we will do the right thing for the future generations of Americans.

Nobel prize winners and other scientists,[d] who have dedicated their lives to medical research, agree that animal research is absolutely necessary. Why should we disbelieve these knowledgeable people? Instead, we listen to movie stars who know nothing about science or medicine. Playing a doctor in a movie or on a soap opera, doesn't make them science experts, yet many people are persuaded by their uninformed, misguided, emotional pleas.

The issue is not about humane treatment. Everyone is for the humane treatment of research animals. Universities and government research centers have strict rules that protect all test subjects, animal or human, from mistreatment. The American Veterinary Medical Association supplies qualified veterinarians to care for research animals and enforce federal regulations designed to protect them from abuse. The rare mistreatments of the past are no longer tolerated by the watchful scientific community.

Once a research project is complete, scientists must submit their findings to other scientists from around the world. This prevents studies with no scientific importance from being done.

Sometimes the media will publicize a scientist's work because they know it can be made to sound foolish or needlessly cruel. What the media is really showing is that they are uneducated and uninformed about science.

---

d. Both the American Medical Association (AMA) and the American Veterinary Medical Association (AVMA) agree that animals are vital to continued medical research.

What is the real issue? It's really about medical research—should it continue or be halted? In the Dark Ages, powerful political forces used fear and ignorance to halt the scientific search for truth. Let's not return to those dark times out of our own ignorance. As Albert Einstein once said, "Politics are for the moment. Equations [and discoveries] are forever!"

Thanks to the Animals

Scientists reported in 1991 that research with chimpanzees has led to the discovery of a possible vaccine against HIV. Sixty-five chimpanzees were vaccinated with the experimental vaccine and then injected with live HIV. Chimpanzees were used for the test because they can become HIV positive, but do not get AIDS. This test was repeated several times on the same, vaccinated chimps. It has been over three years since the original test and the animals are still HIV negative!

Jorg Eichberg, Ph.D., the leader of the research team, had this to say about the animals he used to make this important breakthrough: "they deserve our thanks, they contributed to mankind and we are grateful."

Scientists are not monsters who enjoy using animals in their research. Animal research is extremely expensive and involves endless paperwork to receive the necessary permissions. But, medical researchers will tell you that this work is absolutely vital, especially for AIDS research.

The next step for Dr. Eichberg's vaccine is to test it on humans with a high risk for HIV infection. Whether the vaccine will protect people, only time will tell. One thing is for certain: human volunteers will feel much better about using this new vaccine knowing that our animal friends have tried it first.

Using animals to conduct scientific research is not new. In 1890, two scientists working with animals discovered they could produce a substance that prevented diphtheria, a terrible bacterial disease that occurred most often in children.

On Christmas night 1891, a child with diphtheria became the first to receive the medicine. She recovered completely. This experiment was one of the great success stories of medicine. A terrible bacterial disease was finally controlled. Today, this disease is rarely seen.

Since the very beginning of modern medical research, animals have contributed enormously to our knowledge, and have helped to improve medicine. These improvements have increased the average life span from 47.3 years in 1900 to nearly 72 years in 1993! When a cure for AIDS and cancer are discovered, both scientists and animals will be responsible, not well meaning movie and television stars.

Here is a very brief list of only a few of the major accomplishments animals have helped to discover:

- Understanding the aging process and how Alzheimer's disease affects the elderly.

- Chest surgery and lung transplant techniques.[e]

- Development and testing of penicillin.

- Animals opened the way for successful brain surgery on humans.

- Important discoveries about how the human brain works.

- Discovery that the right side of the brain functions differently than the left side.

- Understanding of genetics and inherited diseases.

- Understanding both age-related and work-related hearing loss.[f]

---

e. The first patient with lung cancer to have a lung removed lived for 40 more years thanks to animal research. Every person to have chest surgery of any type has the animals to thank.
f. Helped establish the first workplace noise exposure limits.

- Understanding of behavioral illnesses, such as anorexia and chronic anxiety.

- Research with primates helped develop new approaches to teaching the mentally retarded.

- Discovery of the link between obesity (extreme overweight) and shortened life span.

- The importance of nutrition and which factors are important to improved health.

- The first chemotherapy drugs to combat cancer.

- Identification of environmental factors that cause cancer.

- The discovery that some cancers are caused by viruses.

- Therapies and treatments for breast cancer.

- Future, potential cures for all cancers.

- All techniques for heart surgery— heart repair, transplanting, and artificial hearts.

- Coronary artery bypass surgery and the "heart/lung" machine.

- Development of the "pump oxygenator," a machine used in heart and lung operations.

- Drugs to control heart attacks.

- Development of the heart pacemaker.

- Drugs to control high blood pressure.

- Proved the link between stress and heart disease.

- Found the link between fatty foods and hardening of the arteries (arteriosclerosis).

- Discovered the link between high serum cholesterol and heart diseases.

- A vaccine for polio, chicken pox, influenza, encephalitis (brain infections), and rabies.

- Therapies and prevention of beriberi, smallpox, rubella, cholera, measles, mumps, and diphtheria.

- Understanding and treatment of epilepsy.

- Discovery and testing of insulin to control diabetes.

- Understanding and treatment of ulcers.

- Treatments for hemophilia.

- Discovery that bone marrow transplants can cure certain blood disorders.

- Therapy for hepatitis infections.

- The world's first hepatitis B vaccine.

- Studying the link between alcohol and liver disease (cirrhosis).

- Treatment and potential new therapies for malaria.[g]

- Study and development of therapies for muscular dystrophy.

- Treatments for eye diseases, including glaucoma and cataracts.

- Understanding of how the brain and eye communicate.

- Treatment of children's eye disorders.

- First successful transplant of liver, heart, lung, and other organs.

- Discovery of the cause for Parkinson's disease.

- Discovery of how tuberculosis (TB) is transmitted.

Without question, we owe a lot to our animal friends. They have helped us to eliminate much needless suffering, pain, and grief. Without them, most of what we have learned would have remained undiscovered.

For this reason, this book is dedicated to the animals. They have aided us in the quest for a world without diseases, sickness, or illness. We owe the animals a great deal. Many children, women, and men owe them their very lives. Look

g. Malaria affects 200 million people worldwide.

over the previous list once more and you'll probably find that you owe them a thank you, too.

Besides the animal rights activists, another group of people are striving to end all animal research. They are scientists whose mission is to discover new ways to perform research and test new medicines without the use of animals. Today this is still an impossible dream, but it is a goal that all scientists and doctors hope to achieve one day.

Someday we won't raise animals for food, turn their fur and feathers into clothing, or make boots, shoes, car seats, and glue out of their hides. No one will hunt or trap wild creatures of any type. No one will go fishing. We won't eat hamburger, *Jell-O®*, or bacon. And someday scientists and doctors will discover a better way to do the research desperately needed to wipe out diseases and save lives. You can be sure when this day finally comes, no one will rejoice more than the scientists who made it possible.

❏ FAST TRACK

1. Researchers are making discoveries that will ultimately lead to the cure of all diseases caused by viruses.

2. The FDA is responsible for approving all new drugs in the United States.

3. A number of important drugs have been approved to combat HIV, but none are a cure.

4. The FDA is testing about 400 new drugs for safety and effectiveness.

5. Thanks to AIDS activist groups and doctors, the FDA is quicker about approving drugs for experimental use on humans.

6. The easiest way to stop the spread of HIV is with a safe and effective vaccine.

7. At least eight vaccines are currently being studied in limited human testing.

8. Researchers are looking for vaccines that make the immune system produce massive amounts of antibodies to fight HIV.

9. The deadly smallpox virus was eliminated thanks to a worldwide vaccination program.

10. Researchers must prove that a potential vaccine is safe and will not cause dangerous side effects.

11. Vaccines must completely protect the vaccinated person.

12. A successful vaccine must stop all strains or types of HIV.

13. A mixture or "cocktail" of different drugs may prove to be the most effective vaccine.

14. It can cost tens of millions of dollars to get approval for a prescription drug. Years of research and millions of dollars can be spent only to discover the drug makes humans too sick.

15. All new medicines and breakthrough medical procedures must first be tested to determine if they are safe.

16. A vaccine or cure for HIV/AIDS will never be discovered without the help of animals.

17. Americans frequently hear distorted or incomplete stories from the media. Being responsible members of society, we should get all the facts before we make hasty judgments.

18. Nobel prize winners and other scientists agree that animal research is absolutely necessary.

19. Everyone is for the humane treatment of research animals.

20. Universities and government research centers have strict rules designed to protect all test subjects, animal or human, from mistreatment.

21. The American Veterinary Medical Association supplies qualified veterinarians to care for research animals and enforce federal regulations designed to protect them from abuse.

❏ TEST YOUR KNOWLEDGE

Answers are in Appendix B.

1. The _____ is responsible for approving all new drugs in the United States.

2. A _____ would prevent the spread of HIV to un-infected people.

3. Although HIV prefers to infect _____
   _____ _____, other types of cells are also infected.

4. _____ is for the humane treatment of research animals.

5. The American Veterinary Medical Association supplies qualified _____ to care for research animals and enforce federal regulations designed to protect them from abuse.

6–9. List four important discoveries that could not have been made without animal research.

10. True or False

   According to chapter 5, all scientists are cruel, unfeeling brutes who care nothing about humane treatment of animals.

❏ REFERENCE NOTES

1. Frakelmann, K. (1991, October). Survival bonus for people with AIDS. *Science News, 140,* p. 260.

2. *JAMA, 266* (6), (1991, August 14), p. 763.

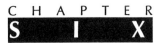

Hepatitis

Hepatitis is a serious disease with many causes. Hepatitis is actually a general term describing any infection or inflammation (swelling) of the liver. Hepatitis lasting for several weeks or months is called *acute hepatitis* (acute meaning short term). *Chronic hepatitis* is inflammation that lasts longer than six months (chronic meaning long term).

A variety of things causes hepatitis—alcohol or drug abuse, overexposure to certain chemicals, prescription medication, even herbal medicines, teas, and tonics. However, hepatitis is most commonly caused by a virus infection in the liver.

Viral Hepatitis

Hepatitis has been around for a long time. Hippocrates, "the Father of Medicine," described epidemics of hepatitis almost 25 centuries ago.

There are five types of hepatitis known to be caused by virus infections.[a] These various types of hepatitis range in symptoms, severity, and long-term health effects. Some are

---

a. A sixth type (hepatitis F) is suspected to exist, but has not been identified.

short lived and do not pose serious health threats; other types can cause permanent damage and death.

The five types of viral hepatitis infections are named after the letters of the alphabet—hepatitis A, hepatitis B, hepatitis C, hepatitis D, and hepatitis E.[b] Like HIV, hepatitis viruses are parasites that must infect a host cell.

Although, HIV/AIDS gets most of the media's attention, viral hepatitis is a more serious threat to the general public. Certain types of hepatitis are 100 times more infectious than HIV.[1]

As with HIV, the media also exaggerates information about hepatitis. Magazines frequently report that 700,000 cases of viral hepatitis occur each year. The truth is, no one knows how many cases occur each year, but most experts agree that 300,000–500,000 is more realistic. Most cases are very mild and produce no symptoms. Probably only 1 in 10 cases ever gets reported.[2]

Even without the exaggerations, hepatitis is a potentially serious disease. In 1993, 42,115 Americans reported hepatitis infections.[3] During the first 11 years of the AIDS epidemic over 600,000 people in the United States reported hepatitis infections. As many as five million more cases may have gone unreported.

Unlike AIDS, viral hepatitis is not always life threatening. Still, it can cause chronic (long-term) illness, as well as death.

The first symptoms of hepatitis infections are typically fever, nausea, stomach pain, loss of appetite, achiness, and constant fatigue. Sometimes, the urine turns brown, but more often, the white parts of the eyes become yellow, as if stained by a dye. The skin also takes on a yellow color.

Jaundice, or yellowing of the eyes and skin, often occurs in hepatitis. Jaundice is a symptom, not a disease. Jaundice

---

b. Type C was previously named hepatitis non-A, non-B.

can be a sign of several diseases or disorders in the body.[c] It is caused by a build up of a pigment called **bilirubin.** As the pigment builds up in tissue, the skin and eyes develop a yellow discoloration. Normal livers quickly break down bilirubin. Hepatitis infections slow down this process, allowing the pigment to accumulate.

Hepatitis can be highly contagious. Studies show that health care workers who accidentally stick themselves with HIV-contaminated needles have a 0.3% chance of becoming infected. But, health care workers who stick themselves with hepatitis-infected needles run a 30% chance of being infected.[4]

Hepatitis viruses prefer to infect liver cells. In the case of chronic viral hepatitis, the virus may live indefinitely in the person's liver. When this happens, the infected person may recover from the illness but will remain infected for life. **Carriers** show no outward symptoms of infection, but carry the virus and can infect others.

Hepatitis A

In 1992, a total of 21,009 cases of hepatitis A were reported. (As mentioned before, many cases go unreported.) Hepatitis A was 48.5% of all reported viral hepatitis infections in 1992. In any given year, about 10 people per 100,000 become infected with hepatitis A. Increased numbers of cases are usually seen in areas where sanitation is poorest.

Hepatitis A is the least dangerous type. It is spread by eating or drinking food and water contaminated with feces. It is often transmitted in restaurants by infected food handlers who do not wash their hands after using the rest room. Outbreaks have also occurred from eating seafood caught in sewage-contaminated water.

---

c. Jaundice is sometimes seen in newborn children, but with treatment it usually disappears quickly.

Hepatitis A is commonly called *infectious hepatitis.* The virus spreads easily to others, usually family members or those living in close quarters with an infected person. Normally, hepatitis A causes symptoms within 15 to 40 days after exposure. Many people become infected and never show symptoms or feel ill. Blood tests have revealed hepatitis antibodies in many individuals who were never diagnosed with the illness.

There is no treatment, but the person usually recovers fully with no long-term damage to the health. This virus does not continue to live in the body after infection; therefore, no one becomes a hepatitis A carrier.

During the summer of 1992, clinical trials on a new vaccine for type A hepatitis were carried out. These trials proved to be 100% successful, but the vaccine will not be commercially available until 1994.[5]

As with all hepatitis infections, drinking of alcoholic beverages should be avoided. The liver is not functioning properly, and alcohol can cause it to be overworked and further damaged.

Hepatitis B

Hepatitis B is one of the more serious types of viral liver infections. The virus that causes hepatitis B is very different from the one that causes hepatitis A. Hepatitis B infection is often called *serum hepatitis* (Figure 6-1). It used to be transmitted mainly through blood transfusions and in other blood products.

In the early sixties the risk of contracting hepatitis from a blood transfusion in the United States was about 33% (1 in 3). Now, routine blood screen has lowered the risk to about 5% (1 in 20).[6] Before routine testing, transfusion-related hepatitis infections caused between 1,500 and 3,000 deaths per year.[7] This number has now been reduced by 90% thanks to regular testing of all donated blood.

FIGURE 6–1

The blood of a person infected with hepatitis B. The round objects are hepatitis B virus particles (highly magnified by an electron microscope). *(From: VIRUSES by A.J. Levine. Copyright © 1991 by W.H. Freeman and Company. Reprinted by permission.)*

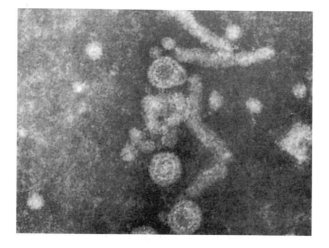

In 1992, 34% of all reported cases of hepatitis were caused by the type B virus. Experts believe that 100,000 to 200,000 cases may go unreported. But remember, these are estimates. The actual number could be much lower and probably not higher.

Today, hepatitis B is transmitted in the exact same ways as HIV. Most new infections are traced to sharing needles, anal and vaginal sex, and from mother to newborn. (Infections spread from a mother to her newborn child are called **vertical transmission**.) Hepatitis B is many times more infectious than HIV. Although HIV is not spread by kissing, hepatitis B **can be transmitted in saliva**. Usually, those who are at risk for HIV infections are even more likely to be infected by hepatitis B virus.

The incubation period for this virus is 60–160 days. At first, most people report symptoms similar to those caused by hepatitis A—fever, aches, nausea, stomach pain, loss of appetite, fatigue, and yellow eyes and skin. The majority develop acute hepatitis that may last for several months. The acute form may cause permanent liver damage and only very rarely death. Infected people will usually recover fully.

The disease is more devastating to babies infected by vertical transmission. Their immune systems are not fully developed, so about 80% of infected infants develop chronic or long-term disease. Sadly, 25% of these babies will die of chronic liver disease by the time they are adults.[8] Children that escape infection from their mothers at birth remain at high risk for the first five years of life. Preventative vaccinations after birth could prevent most of these children from developing infections later in life.

Approximately 10% of adults infected with hepatitis B virus become chronic, lifetime carriers. Long-term infection of the liver leads to *cirrhosis* or permanent liver scarring. Liver damage occurs when killer T cells (chapter 3) attack the virus and infected liver cells.

In carriers, the virus lives in the liver. After 30–50 years of infection, these people often develop a liver cancer called *HCC (hepatocellular carcinoma)*. The hepatitis B virus is the second most dangerous known cancer-causing agent in humans.[9] Only tobacco products cause more cancers.

Worldwide, there are an estimated 300 million carriers of hepatitis B, but 75% of these are in Asia alone and many more are in Africa. In the United States and Europe, less than 1% of the population are chronic carriers.

Recently, a vaccine that prevents hepatitis B infection was developed. The World Health Organization (WHO) now vaccinates these "hot spots" of infection. Hopefully, the disease will at last be controlled, especially in third world countries where 10% or more of the population are chronic carriers. A trial vaccination program among native Alaskans resulted in a 99% decrease in hepatitis B infections.

Hepatitis C

Until recently, this virus was called non-A/non-B hepatitis. All that was known was that it was neither the A nor the B variety. In 1989, scientists at the Chiron Corporation, a small genetic engineering laboratory in California, discovered the hepatitis C virus.

As mentioned before, the viruses that cause types A and B hepatitis are very different from each other. The same is true for type C hepatitis virus. Each of these viruses comes from completely different families, but they have one thing in common—they all prefer to infect liver cells.

Although there are many estimates about the number of hepatitis C cases that occur each year, no one really knows for certain. There are definitely fewer infections of this type than the A or B virus. Although the popular press claims that hepatitis C accounts for as much as 33% of all hepatitis in the United States, more responsible authorities say that it is actually around 3%.[10]

Hepatitis C is a serious illness, but much is still not understood. It can cause both acute and chronic disease and has also been linked to chronic liver disease and cancer. The incubation period is unclear. It can be as short as a few weeks or as long as one year.

How this virus is transmitted is also unclear. Over half of the known cases are linked to sharing needles, but the remaining cases were transmitted by unknown means. Experts feel that many of the same factors that place a person at risk for HIV and hepatitis B, also contribute to hepatitis C.

Hepatitis B and C viruses accumulate in the blood and saliva in far greater amounts than HIV. This is one reason why these viruses are far more contagious than HIV. They are also potentially fatal.

5. The types of viral hepatitis are named hepatitis A, hepatitis B, hepatitis C, hepatitis D, and hepatitis E.

6. Like HIV, hepatitis viruses must infect a host cell.

7. Certain types of hepatitis are 100 times more infectious than HIV.

8. In 1993, 42,115 Americans were reported infected with hepatitis. Total infections, reported and unreported may be between 300,000 and 500,000.

9. During the first 11 years of the AIDS epidemic over 6 million people were infected with hepatitis.

10. The first symptoms of hepatitis infections are typically fever, nausea, stomach pain, loss of appetite, achiness, constant fatigue, and yellowing of the eyes and skin (jaundice).

11. Jaundice, caused by a build up of a pigment called bilirubin, is a symptom of several diseases or disorders in the body.

12. Normally, the liver quickly breaks down bilirubin, but hepatitis causes it to accumulate.

13. Hepatitis virus prefers to infect liver cells and may remain for life.

14. Carriers show no outward symptoms of infection, but are capable of infecting others.

15. Hepatitis A accounts for about 49% of all viral hepatitis infections and is the least dangerous type. About 10 people per 100,000 become infected with hepatitis A.

16. Increased numbers of cases of hepatitis A are seen in areas where sanitation is poorest.

17. Hepatitis A is spread by eating or drinking food and water contaminated with feces.

18. People infected with hepatitis A do not become carriers.

19. Drinking of alcoholic beverages should be avoided during hepatitis.

20. Hepatitis B, often called serum hepatitis, is one of the more serious types of viral liver infections.

21. Routine blood screening has lowered the risk of hepatitis infection from transfusions to about 5% (1 in 20).

22. Hepatitis B is transmitted in the same ways as HIV, but can also be transmitted in saliva.

23. Those who are at risk for HIV infections are more likely to be infected by hepatitis B virus.

24. Long-term infection of the liver leads to cirrhosis or permanent liver scarring.

25. Liver damage occurs when killer T cells attack the virus and infected liver cells.

26. Hepatitis B virus, the second most dangerous cancer-causing agent in humans, can cause liver cancer after 30–50 years of chronic infection.

27. In the United States and Europe, less than 1% of the population are chronic carriers.

28. A vaccine that prevents hepatitis A and B infection has been developed.

29. Trial vaccinations of native Alaskans decreased hepatitis B infections by 99%.

30. Each type of hepatitis virus is different, but all prefer to infect liver cells.

31. Hepatitis C, which has also been linked to chronic liver disease and cancer, accounts for about 3% of all hepatitis in the United States.

32. Many of the same risk factors for HIV and hepatitis B also contribute to hepatitis C.

33. Hepatitis B and C viruses accumulate in blood and saliva in greater amounts than HIV.

34. Hepatitis viruses are far more contagious than HIV.

35. Hepatitis D occurs only in those already infected with hepatitis B virus.

36. Hepatitis D is relatively rare in Europe and the United States.

37. Hepatitis E does not occur in the United States, unless imported by travelers.

38. Hepatitis E is spread by eating and drinking feces-contaminated food or water.

39. Hepatitis E virus is more dangerous to pregnant women and may cause death.

❏ TEST YOUR KNOWLEDGE

Answers are in Appendix B.

1. Hepatitis is a general term that describes any
_____ or _____ of the liver.

2. Hepatitis lasting for several weeks or months is called
_____ hepatitis.

3. _____ hepatitis is inflammation that lasts longer than six months.

4. Name the types of hepatitis.

5. Which two types of hepatitis are most dangerous in combination with each other?

6. Which types of hepatitis are spread through contaminated food or water?

7. Which type causes the most hepatitis infections in the United States?

8. _____ is caused by a build up of a pigment called bilirubin that causes the skin and eyes to develop a yellow discoloration.

9. List five behaviors that place a person at risk for hepatitis infection.

10. Which types of hepatitis can cause cancer?

❏ REFERENCE NOTES

1. *JAMA, 226* (6), (1991, August 14), p. 771.

2. Personal communication with Dr. Frank Mahoney of the Center for Disease Control.

3. *MMWR, 41* (52 & 53), (1993, January 8).

4. *JAMA, 266* (6), (1991, August 14) p. 771.

5. Organs spread hepatitis C. (1992, August 15). *Science News, 142,* p. 103.

6. *JAMA, 263* (13), (1990, April 4), p. 1749.

7. Levine, Arnold J. (1992). *Viruses,* (p. 181). New York: Scientific American Library.

8. *MMWR, 40* (RR-13), (1991, November 22), p. 3.

9. *Scientific American, 264* (4), (1991, April), p. 116.

10. *JAMA, 263* (13), (1990, April 4), p. 1749.

11. *JAMA, 261* (9), (1989, March 3), p. 1321.

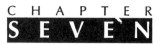

C H A P T E R
SEVEN

Sanitation and Disinfection

Controlling infectious agents is an important part of the salon industry. Clients depend upon you to ensure their safety. Protecting against the spread of infectious organisms is also required by both federal and state regulations and for good reason.

Salon professionals come in contact with many people each day. Your services provide clients with great benefits. However, if proper care is not taken you could contribute to the spread of disease.

The first six chapters of this book provide you with the understanding of infections and diseases. Now let's focus on controlling potentially harmful microorganisms.

Contamination and Decontamination

Look around the room for a moment. What do you see? No matter where you are, you will always see a surface of some sort. The surface of the table, the wall, the floor, your hand—most things have a surface. No matter how clean you keep these surfaces, they will eventually become *contaminated.*

Surfaces of tools or other objects that are not clean or free from microorganisms are contaminated. Substances that cause contamination are called *contaminants.* The contaminating substance can be many things. Hair in a comb or makeup on a towel are contaminants. Hair is not supposed to be in a clean comb, nor is makeup normally found on clean towels.

Tools and other surfaces in the salon can also be contaminated with bacteria, viruses, and fungi. Even clean tools are covered with these microorganisms.

It would be impossible to keep the salon free from all contamination, and it is not necessary to try. Most microorganisms are harmless and coexist with humans without causing problems. Many are actually beneficial. Yeast, for example, is a microorganism that bread lovers and beer drinkers would not care to do without. However, some microorganisms are dangerous and must be kept under strict control.

Microorganisms that cause disease are called *pathogens.* Salon professionals must be on constant alert in order to control pathogens.

Removing harmful organisms or other substances from tools or surfaces is called *decontamination.* There are three main levels of decontamination, but only two of these decontamination levels are useful in the salon.

Sterilization

Sterilization is the most effective type of decontamination. As the name implies, sterilization completely destroys all living organisms on an object or surface. Sterilization even kills bacterial spores, the most resistant form of life on Earth.

Sterilization is the highest of the three levels of decontamination. It is a multistep, time-consuming, and difficult process. Obviously, it is unnecessary, impractical, and virtually impossible to sterilize tools and surfaces in the salon.

The word "sterilize" often is used incorrectly. For example, some practitioners tell clients they are sterilizing the nail plate or skin. This is impossible! Sterilizing the skin would quickly kill it and would certainly destroy the nail plate as well.

It is not important to kill all microorganisms in the salon. Pathogens, the disease-causing organisms, are the real target. Most do not normally exist in the salon, but are carried in by clients or workers.

Sanitization

The lowest level of decontamination is called **sanitation** or **sanitizing.** These words are frequently misused and misunderstood.

Sanitation means to significantly reduce the numbers of pathogens found on a surface. If pathogens are reduced to levels considered safe by public health standards, the object or surface is sanitized. Salon tools and surfaces are sanitized by cleaning with soaps or detergents.

Sanitized surfaces may still have pathogens and other organisms on them. Removing hair from a brush and washing it with detergent is considered sanitation. Putting antiseptics on skin or nail plates is sanitization.

Washing your hands is another example of sanitation. Your hands may be very clean when you are finished, but they are still covered with microorganisms. The tap water and the towel you dried your hands with contain bacteria.

This does not mean that washing your hands is useless or unnecessary. On the contrary! Frequent hand washing is an important way to control the spread of dangerous organisms. The bacteria in water or on the towel are normally harmless in the salon.

By washing your hands, you remove many types of contaminants. Dirt, oils, residue from salon products, as well as pathogens are removed by frequent hand washing. Certain hand sanitizers are designed to be left on the hands after use. Although these products are effective, you will still need to wash your hands frequently. These "leave-on" sanitizers will not remove oils, dirt, and chemical residues.

❑ **Wash Your Hands!**

One in five salon workers will develop a skin disorder during their career. Prolonged or repeated contact to professional products can cause irritation and allergic reactions.

Wash your hands often and remember to dry them thoroughly. When hands are not kept dry, cracked, dry skin, even open sores, can develop.

Hand washing is an important part of your service. Washing prevents spreading potentially dangerous organisms from one client to another.

It is especially important to wash between every client, no matter how busy your day.

Make a ceremony of washing your hands in front of your clients. It is one way of assuring that they will come back again and again.

The Professional Establishment

Sanitation should be a part of every professional's normal routine. In this way, you and your coworkers can maintain a professional-looking establishment. Below are some simple guidelines that will help keep the salon looking its best.

■ Floors should be swept clean whenever needed.

■ Hair, cotton balls, etc. should be picked up immediately.

■ Deposit all waste materials in a metal waste receptacle with a self-closing lid.

- It is important to control all types of dust. Mop floors and vacuum carpets daily.

- Windows, screens, and curtains should be clean.

- All work areas must be well lighted.

- Salons need both hot and cold running water.

- Rest rooms must be clean and tidy.

- Toilet tissue, paper towels, and liquid soap must be provided.

- Wash hands after using the rest room and between clients.

- Clean sinks and drinking fountains regularly.

- Separate or disposable drinking cups must be provided.

- The salon must be free from insects and rodents.

- Salons should never be used for cooking or living quarters.

- Food must never be placed in refrigerators used to store salon products.

- Eating, drinking, and smoking are prohibited in the salon.

- Waste receptacles must be emptied regularly throughout the day.

- Employees must wear clean, freshly washed clothing.

- Always use freshly laundered towels on each client.

- Capes or other covering should not contact client's skin.

- Makeup, lipstick, puffs, pencils, and brushes must never be shared.

- Clean cotton balls or sponges should be used to apply cosmetics and creams.

- Remove products from containers with clean spatulas, not fingers.

of active ingredients, and a list of the viruses and other organisms against which the product is effective. Federal regulations also require that you be provided with one other very important information sheet. This information sheet is called a ***Material Safety Data Sheet*** (MSDS). Federal regulations require each salon to have an MSDS for every professional product that contains a potentially hazardous ingredient.

Don't just toss these information sheets into a drawer or throw them out with the packing material. Special federal laws have been passed to ensure that you are given this vital information. Take the time to read it to be certain you are protecting yourself and clients to the best of your ability (Figure 7–1).

FIGURE 7–1
Read your MSDSs. *(Photo by Michael A. Gallitelli, from* Milady's Art and Science of Nail Technology, *3rd edition, copyright © 1992 by Milady Publishing Company.)*

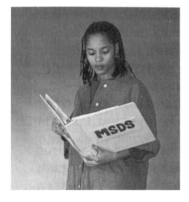

Properly Using Disinfectants

The best way to learn the proper use of disinfectants is to read the manufacturer's instructions. You should also periodically review these directions in case new information is added. Trade shows are another place to learn disease/infection control techniques. Manufacturers will often host special seminars designed to teach you the basics of proper salon disinfection. Watch for them in your area or call the manufacturers listed in Appendix A (page 131–132) for more information.

High-quality disinfectants must perform several special jobs in the salon. They must be **bactericides** (kill harmful bacteria)[a] and **fungicides** (destroy fungi). Disinfectants that perform both of these functions are called **hospital level disinfectants.** This is the highest level of disinfection and exceeds the minimum requirements for salon disinfection.

But even the most advanced, high-tech disinfectants available can't do the job, unless used correctly. Implements should always be thoroughly cleaned before soaking to avoid contaminating the disinfecting solution. Hair, nail filings, creams, oils, and makeup will lessen the effectiveness of the solution.

The jars or containers used to disinfect implements are often incorrectly called **wet sanitizers.** Of course, the purpose of these jars is not to sanitize, but to disinfect. The disinfecting soak solution must be changed daily unless otherwise directed by the manufacturer's instructions.

If implements are sanitized (washed) before disinfecting, the soak solution will be more effective. Some foolishly believe that using dirty or contaminated disinfectant is better than nothing. But if your clients see you pull an implement from a jar of dirty liquid, they will strongly disagree. You'll find they won't be your clients for long.

After the manufacturer's specified period, the disinfectant solution is useless and must be discarded. Control of

---

a. Hospital-strength disinfectants must be effective against *Staphylococcus aureus, Salmonella choleraesuis,* and *Pseudomonas aeruginosa* infectious diseases is one area of the salon where you can't afford to skimp just to save a few pennies.

The EPA recommends that implements be fully immersed for a **minimum** of 10 minutes.

HIV and Tuberculosis Claims

You have learned that it is practically impossible to transmit HIV in the salon. The same is true for tuberculosis (TB). There has never been a case of TB transmission in the salon. Tuberculosis is not transmitted by salon implements; it is spread only by coughing and, in rare instances, contaminated milk.

Many disinfectant systems claim to be effective against both HIV and TB, but these pathogens are not of great concern to salon professionals. Fungi, cold or flu viruses, and infection-causing pathogenic bacteria are many thousands of times more likely to be spread by your implements. In short, don't choose your disinfectants simply because of HIV and TB claims. These marketing claims play on people's fear and have little importance in the salon.

Types of Disinfectants

Quaternary ammonium compounds (quats) are safe and fast acting. Older formulas relied on only one quat, but newer products use blends of several different quats to increase effectiveness.

Most quat solutions disinfect implements in 10 to 15 minutes. Leaving certain implements in for too long may damage them. Long-term exposure to any water solution can damage fine steel.

With today's modern formulas, corrosion of metal surfaces can be easily avoided, especially if you keep implements separated from each other. Still, metal implements such as

❏ Misunderstood Alcohol

Every alcohol is different. Therefore, it is important not to lump all types together as if they were the same.

For example, methyl alcohol is also called wood alcohol, because it is obtained by distilling wood. This type of alcohol is poisonous and causes blindness if ingested.

Methyl alcohol's closest relative is ethyl alcohol, also called grain alcohol. Grain alcohol is obtained by distilling grain and is not nearly as poisonous. In fact, it is the same alcohol found in vodka, beer, and wine.

Isopropyl alcohol (rubbing alcohol) is also very closely related to methyl and ethyl alcohol. It is very poisonous to drink.

Each of these three alcohols is a clear liquid with a strong odor. They are each very flammable and drying to skin and hair. However, this is not true of all alcohols. In fact, only a very few alcohols have these properties.

For example, cetyl alcohol and stearyl alcohol are waxy feeling, white, solid substances. They have practically no odor. They are non-toxic if ingested and are not flammable. They do not dry the skin; in fact, they are both excellent skin and hair conditioners.

Moral—Don't judge an alcohol by its name.

scissors and nail clippers should be oiled regularly to keep them in perfect working order. Quats are also very effective for cleaning table and counter tops.

***Phenols (phenolics)*,** like quats, have been used for many years to disinfect implements. They too can be safe and extremely effective if used according to instructions. Care should be taken to avoid skin contact with phenols. The concentrated liquid can cause skin irritation and some are corrosive, especially to the eyes.

Alcohol is often misunderstood. Actually, there are thousands of types of alcohols. The three most common types are methyl alcohol (methanol), ethyl alcohol (ethanol), and isopropyl alcohol (isopropanol). A general rule of thumb is, a chemical name ending with the letters *ol* indicates the substance is an alcohol.

In the salon, ethyl and isopropyl alcohol are often used for disinfecting implements. To be effective, the strength of ethyl alcohol must be no less than 70%. (The other 30% is water.) Isopropyl alcohol's strength must be 99% or it is ineffective.

There are several disadvantages to using alcohols. They are extremely flammable, evaporate quickly, and are slow-acting, less-effective disinfectants. Alcohols corrode tools and cause sharp edges to become dull. The vapors formed upon evaporation can cause headaches and nausea in high concentrations or after prolonged exposure.

If used at lower than the specified percentage, alcohols are not effective disinfectants. Unfortunately, alcohols absorb water from the air. In areas of high humidity, this is an even greater problem. Also, if the implements are not absolutely dry when added to the alcohol, the water on them can further dilute the solution. The combined effects of absorbing water from the air and water added with implements can quickly destroy the alcohol's ability to disinfect.

Household bleach (sodium hypochlorite) is an effective disinfectant, but shares some of the same drawbacks as alcohols. Neither bleach nor alcohols are professionally designed and tested for disinfection of salon implements. Bleach can also discolor some materials. Bleach was used extensively in the past, but has since been replaced by more advanced and effective technologies.

Although quats are perfectly suitable for cleaning any surface (unless otherwise specified in the manufacturer's directions), you may wish to clean floors, bathrooms, sinks, and waste receptacles, with a commercial cleaner such as Lysol® or Pine Sol® (phenolic cleaners). Both are very effective disinfectants, but **should not be used on salon implements**. They are general, household-level disinfectants and are not designed for implements or other professional tools.

What's Best for the Salon?

With so many product choices and so many conflicting claims, how do you choose the system that is best for your salon? It's easy! Any EPA registered, hospital level disinfectant will provide more than enough protection for normal salon use. Stronger disinfectants are not necessary and in many cases are too dangerous to use in the salon environment.

Some states now require that tuberculocidal disinfectants be used only when visible blood is present. If no visible blood is present on your tools, then tuberculocidal disinfectants are not required. As you know, tuberculosis is NOT spread by implements. However, they are more a little more effective on blood and are recommended to clean up blood spills. If you live in a state with such a regulation, you should keep an extra container filled with a tuberculocidal disinfectant in case you accidentally cut a client.

Ultrasonic Cleaners

Ultrasonic baths are useful when combined with disinfectants. Ultrasonic baths use high frequency sound waves to create bubbles in the solution. These tiny bubbles collapse inwards with great force, creating a powerful cleansing action. This cleansing action is a highly effective way to clean nooks and crannies that are impossible to reach with a brush. Still, without an effective disinfectant solution, these devices will only sanitize implements.

Ultrasonic cleaners are a useful addition to your disinfection process, but are not required equipment. Many systems disinfect with great effectiveness without such devices. However, some feel this added cleaning benefit is well worth the extra expense.

Disinfectant Safety

All disinfectants can be hazardous if used incorrectly. Regardless of manufacturer claims of safety, disinfectants are not to be treated lightly. Disinfectants are powerful, professional-strength tools. Disinfectants of all types are poisonous if ingested. Many can cause skin and eye damage, especially in a concentrated form. Use caution to keep them away from small children.

Don't let these words of warning frighten you away from using disinfectants as a regular part of your routine. If used correctly, professionally formulated disinfectant products are safe. In fact, the consequences you face from not using disinfectants are far more serious. Use them wisely and disinfectants will work for you and your clients.

Other Surfaces

You must consider many other surfaces, for example, table or counter tops, telephone receivers, doorknobs, cabinet handles, mirrors, and cash registers. Any surface can be contaminated, especially if touched by clients and staff. These items must also be sanitized regularly.

Estheticians must disinfect electrodes, attachments, brushes, beds, tweezers, and items used for facials and makeup applications. Nail technicians must disinfect clippers, manicure and foot baths (pedicure bowls), files, buffers, and table tops. Cosmetologists must disinfect mixing utensils, combs, brushes, pins, clips, curlers, hair dryers, and chairs.

Tanning beds must be cleaned and disinfected between each client. Open sores on a client's body can leave contagious viruses behind. The microorganisms that cause herpes and shingles, for example, can be spread in this fashion.

Look around and you will see, there is far more to keeping the salon safe and sanitary than sweeping the floor and wiping up spills.

To decontaminate most surfaces, wash thoroughly with a detergent, then spray or wipe on a disinfectant recommended for the surface. Wipe and spray again, then allow the surface to air dry. Be sure to wear gloves while disinfecting surfaces; if using a spray bottle, take care to avoid inhalation of the mists.

Ultraviolet Ray Sanitizers

Keep in mind that implements must be disinfected, not simply sanitized, between clients. However, once properly disinfected, your tools must be stored where they will remain free from contamination. Ultraviolet (UV) sanitizers are useful storage containers. The ultraviolet rays can kill many kinds of bacteria, but they **will not disinfect salon implements.** UV light rays cannot reach into every crevice and are ineffective against viruses. UV sanitizers should be used with care and in strict accordance with manufacturer's instructions. Never use these devices to disinfect!

If you do not wish to use a UV cabinet, you may wrap your implements in clean plastic wrap or seal them in an airtight container.

Electric or Bead Sterilizers

These devices are appropriately named because the only thing they really sterilize are the glass beads inside the unit. They do **not** sterilize implements. They can't even properly disinfect tools. They only give users a dangerously false sense of security.

To effectively sterilize an implement with dry heat, the tools must be heated to 325°F for at least 30 minutes. Effective disinfection can only occur if the entire implement, including handle, is submerged. These devices are a waste of money and a dangerous gamble with your client's health.

Sometimes, UV ray sanitizers and bead sterilizers are sold as FDA-registered devices. FDA registration can be very misleading and usually means very little to salon professionals. A device can be registered as a sanitizer and then deceptively sold as a disinfection unit. In short, don't buy anything simply because it is "FDA registered."

Antiseptics

Antiseptics can kill bacteria and slow their growth, but they are not disinfectants. Antiseptics are weaker than disinfectants and are safe for application to skin. They are considered to be on the level of sanitizers and should never be used on implements.

Beware of Formalin

For many years, **formalin** has been recommended as a disinfectant and fumigant in dry cabinet sanitizers. Formalin can be purchased as a liquid solution or in tablet form. Although formalin is effective, **it is not safe for salon use**.

The gas released from formalin tablets or liquid is called **formaldehyde.** Formaldehyde is a suspected human cancer-causing agent.[1] It is poisonous to inhale or touch and is very irritating to the eyes, nose, throat, and lungs. It can also cause skin irritation, dryness, and rash.

Formaldehyde is also a strong **allergic sensitizer.** Prolonged or repeated exposure can cause allergic reactions similar to chronic bronchitis or asthma. These symptoms usually worsen over time with continued exposure. These allergic symptoms usually do not appear until after several months or years of use. Practitioners who have become accustomed to using formalin don't suspect it as the source of these health problems.

Salon Safety

Be sure to read and exactly follow the instructions provided with any professional salon product. Wear gloves and safety glasses when mixing and using any products, including disinfectants. Disposable, powdered latex gloves work best. They are discarded after each use. Old, worn out rubber gloves can become a source of contamination themselves. Your skin is a barrier between you and microorganisms. Keep that barrier healthy and intact by wearing gloves.

Both gloves and safety glasses serve as barriers between you and the world around you. These barriers can prevent microorganisms from entering your body through broken skin, hang nails, irritated or dry, scaly areas.

Never pour alcohol, quats, phenols, or any other disinfectant over your hands. This foolish practice can cause skin disease and increase the chance of infection. Wash your hands with an antiseptic soap or detergent and dry them thoroughly.

Carefully weigh and measure all products to assure they perform at their peak efficiency. Never place any product or other chemical in an unmarked bottle. This is an invitation to accidents and could have disastrous consequences.

Always use tongs or a draining basket to remove implements from wet sanitizers. Store all professional products away from food and in a cool, dark, dry location. Also, be sure they are in a tightly closed container.

Universal Sanitation

Protecting yourself and your clients requires you to do many things. You must use gloves and safety glasses, disinfectants and detergents, personal hygiene and salon cleanliness. When all of these things are performed together, it is called *universal sanitation.*

Universal sanitation must be a concerted effort. You must do all of these things in order to create a safe haven for your clients and coworkers.

Your Professional Responsibility

You have several responsibilities as a salon professional. You have the responsibility to protect your clients from harm. They depend on your training and expertise. Today, clients are more concerned than ever about safety and health issues. No matter how skillfully you perform your services, you cannot expect to be successful unless you are sensitive to these concerns.

You also have a responsibility to yourself. You must protect your health and safety, as well. Don't take shortcuts when it comes to sanitation and disinfection. These important measures are designed to protect you, too!

Also, take time to thoroughly read and understand all manufacturers' directions and precautions for use. It is important and will ensure that you are keeping pace with this fast-moving industry.

Finally, you have a responsibility to your profession. When anyone acts unprofessionally in the salon, everyone's image is tarnished. Clients expect to see you act in a professional manner. This is how trust and respect are earned.

It's All Up To You!

Think about what your clients will see and hear when they visit your salon. Will they find hair and dust in the corner? A messy rest room? Dingy towels and stained capes? Pretend for a moment that you are the client. What would you think if you walked into a poorly maintained or unsanitary salon?

It is also important to pay attention to what client's hear. They need to be reassured that your salon is safe and sanitary. Point out the positive things that you do. Show the clients how you disinfect and explain why. Be proud of your knowledge and skill.

Explain to them the difference between sanitizing and disinfecting. Don't tell them you disinfect to prevent AIDS or TB; tell them you disinfect to ensure their safety. Besides, as discussed in previous chapters, HIV and TB are not problems in the salon.

Be positive in your manner, outlook, and actions. You will find that clients will respect you and feel comfortable in your care. These things are important, no matter where you live, no matter what your specialty. This is being responsible. This is what makes you a professional.

❏ FAST TRACK

1. Controlling infectious agents is an important part of the salon industry.
2. Protection against infectious organisms is required by federal and state regulations.
3. Surfaces of tools or other objects that are not clean are contaminated.
4. Substances that cause contamination are called contaminants.
5. Tools and other surfaces can be contaminated with bacteria, viruses, and fungi.
6. It is impossible to keep the salon free from all contamination, and it is not necessary to try.
7. Microorganisms that cause disease are called pathogens.
8. Removing harmful organisms or other substances from tools or other surfaces is called decontamination.

9. There are three main levels of decontamination—sterilization, disinfection, and sanitation.

10. Sterilization completely destroys all living organisms on an object or surface. It is the highest of the three levels of decontamination, but is unnecessary, impractical, and virtually impossible to accomplish in the salon.

11. The lowest level of decontamination is called sanitation or sanitizing.

12. Sanitation means to significantly reduce the numbers of pathogens to levels considered safe by public health standards.

13. Frequent hand washing is an important way to control the spread of pathogens.

14. Disinfection controls microorganisms on nonliving surfaces. It is the second level of decontamination, a higher level than sanitation and second only to sterilization.

15. Disinfectants are substances that disinfect tools and nonliving surfaces.

16. Disinfectants are not for use on human skin, hair, or nails, and may be irritating to skin with prolonged or repeated contact.

17. All disinfectants must be approved by the EPA and each individual state.

18. A disinfectant's label must also have an EPA registration number.

19. Federal regulations require that you receive a Material Safety Data Sheet (MSDS) for every professional product that contains a potentially hazardous ingredient.

20. The best way to learn to use disinfectants is to read the manufacturer's instructions.

21. Implements should always be precleaned to avoid contaminating the disinfecting solution.

22. Disinfectant solutions should be changed according to manufacturer's instructions.

23. Quaternary ammonium compounds (quats) and phenols are examples of safe and fast-acting disinfectants.

24. There are thousands of types of alcohols, but the three most common types are methyl alcohol (methanol), ethyl alcohol (ethanol), and isopropyl alcohol (isopropanol).

25. To be effective, ethyl alcohol's strength must be no less than 70%.

26. To be effective, isopropyl alcohol's strength must be no less than 99%.

27. There are several disadvantages to using alcohols.

28. Household bleach (sodium hypochlorite) is an effective disinfectant.

29. Bleach and alcohols are not professionally designed disinfection systems.

30. Tanning beds must be cleaned with disinfectants between each client.

31. Ultraviolet (UV) sanitizers are not effective against viruses.

32. Electric or bead sterilizers are not effective ways of disinfecting.

33. Antiseptics can kill bacteria and slow their growth, but they are not disinfectants.

34. Antiseptics are weaker than disinfectants and are designed to be safely applied to skin.

35. Formalin releases formaldehyde and is not safe for salon use.

36. Formaldehyde is a suspected human cancer-causing agent that is poisonous to inhale or touch; irritating to the eyes, nose, throat, and lungs; and can cause skin irritation, dryness, and rash.

37. Formaldehyde is a strong allergic sensitizer.

38. Wear gloves and safety glasses when mixing and using any product.

39. Your hands are barriers between you and microorganisms. Keep that barrier healthy and intact by wearing gloves.

40. Carefully weigh, measure, and label all products.

41. Store all professional products away from food and in a cool, dark, dry location.

❏ TEST YOUR KNOWLEDGE

Answers are in Appendix B.

1. Removing harmful organisms or other substances from tools is called _____.

2. Define sanitation.

3. Disinfectants must never be used on human _____, _____, or _____.

4. Disinfectants must have an ____ _____ number.

5. What is the difference between antiseptics and disinfectants?

6. Name three reasons why formalin is dangerous to use as a disinfectant or sanitizer.

7. Are all microorganisms dangerous to humans?

8. Define pathogen.

9. What should you do to keep disinfectant soak solutions from being quickly contaminated?

10. List ten areas of the salon that require frequent attention to maintain a professional-looking establishment.

❏ REFERENCE NOTES

1. Lewis, R. J., Sr. (1991). *Hazardous Chemicals in the Workplace* (p. 100). New York: Van Nostrand Rheinhold.

A

Important Resource Telephone Numbers

HIV/AIDS Information Hotlines

- American Foundation for AIDS Research
  1-800-392-6327

- American Liver Foundation (Hepatitis)
  1-800-223-0179

- National AIDS Hotline (Center for Disease Control)
  1-800-342-AIDS

- National AIDS Hotline in Spanish
  1-800-344-7432

- National Gay Task Force
  1-800-221-7044

- National Sexually Transmitted Disease Hotline
  1-800-227-8922

- Project Inform (AIDS treatment information)
  1-800-822-7422

Disinfection and Sanitization

- Hakari Products, Inc.
  1-800-255-2705

- Micro-Aseptic Products, Inc.
  1-708-358-6303

- Ultronics
  1-800-262-6262

- Isabel Cristina
  1-800-247-4130

Trade Organizations and Associations

- Aestheticians International Association, Inc.
  1-800-950-8707

- American Beauty Association (ABA)
  1-312-644-6610

- Nail Technicians America
  1-314-534-7980

- Nail Industry Association
  1-800-326-2457

- National Cosmetology Association (NCA)
  1-314-543-7980

Safety Equipment

- Lab Safety Supply
  1-800-356-2501

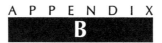

Answers to Test-Your-Knowledge Questions

Chapter 1

1. 1981
2. acquired immune deficiency syndrome
3. HIV, human immunodeficiency virus
4. Central Africa
5. perspective
6. 0.1
7. 1.7
8. True

Chapter 2

1. Cells
2. organisms
3. DNA
4. parasites/host
5. bacteria
6. blood/blood
7. Sharing needles or syringes and anal sex
8. falling/rising

9. 20 million

10. zero

Chapter 3

1. The immune system

2. By the protein overcoat

3. mutate

4. Helper T

5. It has no DNA. It needs a host cell so it can alter the host cell's DNA and force it to make more HIV.

6. Vaccines

7. EIA

8. clear portion of the blood called the serum

9. Western blot test

10. Window/3/6

Chapter 4

1. The immune system

2. Opportunistic

3. Lymph glands

4. Pneumonia (PCP), Kaposi's sarcoma, thrush

5. syndrome

6. True

7. No

8. No

9. No. That is discrimination.

Chapter 5

1. FDA

2. vaccine

3. helper T cells

4. Everyone

5. veterinarians

6–9. See list on pages 89–91 for answers.

10. False

Chapter 6

1. infection/inflammation

2. acute (short-term) hepatitis

3. Chronic

4. hepatitis A, hepatitis B, hepatitis C, hepatitis D, and hepatitis E

5. B and D

6. A and E

7. A

8. Jaundice

9. 1. Direct contact with chronic carriers or their blood

   2. Receiving blood or blood products, as in transfusions

   3. Injecting drugs and sharing needles

   4. Sex with homosexuals or prostitutes

   5. Traveling in foreign countries where hepatitis is prevalent

   6. Working with patients in a hospital (health care workers)

10. B and C

Chapter 7

1. decontamination

2. It is the lowest level of decontamination. Sanitation means to significantly reduce the numbers of patho-

gens from a surface to levels considered safe by public health standards.

3. skin/nails/hair

4. EPA registration

5. Antiseptics can kill bacteria and slow their growth, but they are not as powerful as disinfectants. Antiseptics are weaker and are designed to be safely applied to skin.

6. Formaldehyde, the gas released by formalin tablets or liquid, is a suspected human cancer-causing agent. It is poisonous to inhale or touch and is very irritating to the eyes, nose, throat, and lungs. It can also cause skin irritation, dryness, and rash and is a strong allergic sensitizer. Prolonged or repeated exposure can cause allergic reactions similar to chronic bronchitis or asthma. These symptoms usually worsen over time with continued exposure.

7. No. Most microorganisms are harmless. They coexist with humans without causing problems. Many are actually beneficial.

8. A pathogen is a microorganism that causes disease in humans.

9. Prewash or sanitize implements before disinfecting.

10. See list on pages 113–114 for answers.

Glossary/Index

that is poisonous and may be a carcinogen, 124

Formalin, sanitizing solution that releases formaldehyde gas, 124

Foscarnet, *see* Foscavir

Foscavir, drug used to treat cytomegalovirus eye infections in AIDS sufferers; also called Foscarnet, 82

Flu, 2, 32, 34

Fluconazole, *see* Diflucan

Full-blown AIDS, final stage of AIDS, characterized by multiple infections, which may require extended hospitalization, 74

Fungi, 117, 118

Fungicide, disinfectant that destroys fungi, 117

G

Gancyclovir, *see* Cytovene

Gastroenteritis, viral, often fatal type of diarrhea, 16

Genetic code, arrangement of amino acids in DNA that determine physical characteristics, 28

Genital warts, 40

Glass beads, 123

Glasses, safety, 125

Gloves, as a precaution, 125

Gonorrhea, 40

Government predictions about AIDS, 10

H

Hahn, Beatrice, 4

Hakari Products, 131

Hand washing, 111–112

HCC, hepatocellular carcinoma, a type of liver cancer caused by the hepatitis B virus, 100

Hepatocellular carcinoma, *see* HCC

Helper T cells, immune system cells that instigate an immune response, 56, 58–61, 64, 85

Hepatitis, any infection or swelling of the liver, 32, 40, 47, 95, 96–97, 102
  A type, 97, 98, 101
  acute, lasting only a short period, 95
  B type, 98, 101–102
  C type, 101
  children and, 100
  chronic, prolonged, lasting more than six months, 95
  D type, 102
  E type, 102
  F type, 95
  incubation period, 99
  viral, caused by a virus, 95, 96

Herpes, 123

Herpes simplex, virus associated with cold sores and biologically similar to the HIV virus, 40, 72

Herpes zoster, virus associated with shingles, 72

Hippocrates, 95

HIV, human immunodeficiency virus, the virus that causes AIDS (cf.), xiii, 2
  fragile virus, 35
  geography of, 38
  heterosexual risks, 38
  lifestyles and, 39
  mandatory testing, 65
  multiple exposures, 36
  origin, 3